Sports Injuries
A Self-Help Guide

Second Edition

Vivian Grisogono

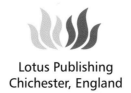

Lotus Publishing
Chichester, England

First published in 1984 by John Murray (Publishers) Ltd. This second edition published in 2012 by Lotus Publishing, Apple Tree Cottage, Inlands Road, Nutbourne, Chichester, West Sussex, PO18 8RJ, UK.

Anatomical Drawings Peter Gardiner
Line Drawings Emily Evans
Text Design Wendy Craig
Cover Design Jim Wilkie
Printed and Bound in the UK by Scotprint

The moral right of the author has been asserted.

MEDICAL DISCLAIMER: The material contained in this book is intended for general reference purposes only. Individuals should always see their health care provider before administering any of the suggestions made. Any application of the material set forth in the following pages is at the reader's discretion and is his or her sole responsibility.

British Library Cataloguing in Publication Data
A CIP record for this book is available from the British Library
ISBN 978 1 905367 28 3

For patient queries and practitioner communications, Vivian Grisogono can be contacted on www.viviangrisogono.com

Contents

"The power of the human body to heal itself is awesome."

Dedication
Dedicated, with thanks, to my family, friends, colleagues and patients.

1

Injuries and Diagnosis

Injuries put you out. This book aims to help you recognize and deal with physical problems which occur through sport or everyday activities. It explains:

- what injuries are and how they happen;
- complications of injury;
- how you can help your doctor or practitioner make an accurate diagnosis;
- what you can do to help yourself;
- how rehabilitation works;
- which exercises are suitable for different injuries.

The information and advice are not substitutes for professional help. For any injury which prevents you from carrying out your normal activities you should consult a professional practitioner. If you are given advice which conflicts with the suggestions in this book, you must accept the word of the person treating you, or seek a further opinion through your doctor.

Types of injury

Physical injuries can be classified into two main groups, traumatic and overuse, and further categorized as extrinsic and intrinsic.

Traumatic injuries

Accidents happen suddenly, and there are immediate effects – perhaps pain, swelling or bleeding. Disorientation and shock can follow shortly afterwards if the accident is serious enough.

Traumatic injuries can happen in two ways: an extrinsic traumatic injury has a recognizable cause, such as a blow, kick or fall; an intrinsic traumatic injury is equally sudden, but its cause is not immediately apparent. A typical example is an Achilles tendon rupture (p. 76), which can occur seemingly out of the blue.

There are three phases in a traumatic injury: the acute phase just after the injury has happened, which lasts a few days; the subacute phase, from about ten days up to four or six weeks; and the chronic phase, when the injury is long-standing and lasts for weeks, months or even longer. In the acute phase the initial pain can be severe, settling quite quickly, or there is little pain at first, but it may increase over the following hours. Through all the phases, the amount and type of pain are often affected by your posture and activities, as well as the degree of damage and inflammation. Very often there is a throbbing feeling. There may or may not be pain at night or when the injured area is at rest.

Sports which involve explosive movements, contact, speed and the possibility of falling or getting hit can give rise to trauma. Such sports include racket games, sprinting, hurdling, steeplechasing, pole vaulting, soccer, American football, rugby, handball, basketball, baseball, cricket, volleyball, field hockey, lacrosse, water polo, karate, tae kwon do, boxing, judo, wrestling, cycle-racing, trampolining, roller blading, skateboarding, horse riding, rock climbing, hang gliding, motor racing, skiing, ice skating, ice hockey and gymnastics.

First aid
Basic first aid should be part of general education. Health professionals, sports coaches and PE teachers in many countries are required to have annual certificates in first aid and life-saving. Life-threatening accidents are rare, but when they happen you need to respond quickly.

As well as recognizing which accidents should be treated as emergencies, every adult involved in sport should be able to deal with minor injuries at any time. A sports kitbag should always include basic first-aid items, especially for dealing with cuts and bruises.

Overuse injuries

Overuse or misuse injuries are intrinsic. They happen through overdoing a particular sport or repetitive activity, poor technique, fatigue, dehydration, excessive heat or cold, or inappropriate equipment. Typical examples include shinbone stress fracture (p. 89), 'shin splints' (p. 90), 'tennis elbow' (p. 279) and 'runner's knee' (p. 103). Overuse injuries are most associated with sports involving repetitive movements, such as running, rowing, canoeing, swimming and cycling, but almost any sport can give rise to overuse, including racket games, throwing events, cricket, golf, fencing, archery, baseball, handball, water polo, sailing, pole vaulting, gymnastics, powerlifting and tug-of-war.

Overuse injuries usually start gradually, which is known technically as 'insidious onset'. There is no acute phase. The first sign is pain felt during or after the activity, perhaps at night or the following morning. If you continue the activity which has caused the problem, the pain gradually gets worse and eventually you have to stop. After a few days' rest you may think the problem has gone, but it returns quickly if you restart your sport without having resolved it.

If an overuse injury is allowed to develop to a chronic phase, the pain increases and starts to interfere with other movements or activities besides the one which caused it. In the case of a stress fracture the bone will not heal if you keep trying it out too soon, and there is a risk that the bone might break altogether.

Injury signs and symptoms

Clinical signs are the injury effects which can be seen or judged objectively, such as bleeding, bruising, swelling, skin colour changes, limited joint movement, muscle wasting (atrophy) and broken bones. They show up when a practitioner examines the injured area, or through diagnostic tests such as X-rays, scans, arthrograms or blood tests.

Injury symptoms are more subjective, although they may overlap with the objective signs. Symptoms are what you feel in the injured area, which may be tingling, numbness, stiffness, temperature changes or pain.

Two important effects of injury are pain and swelling.

Pain

Pain is a warning that something is wrong in the body. Its technical name is 'nociception', meaning your awareness of an unpleasant sensation. Pain is not an accurate guide as to what has happened, or how bad an injury might be. Pain nerves are arranged to function in complex ways. Where you feel the pain is not necessarily where the damage is.

The surface layers of the skin are more sensitive than the deepest layers, so a superficial cut, burn or ligament tear is often more painful than an injury which penetrates more deeply. Pain nerves spread out so that different tissues are served by the same nerve. This means that a problem in one part of the body can transmit pain to another part. This is called 'referred pain'. For instance, injuring your lower back can cause sciatica (p. 219), while a whiplash injury in the neck can transmit symptoms down your arm (p. 227).

People react differently to pain and have different pain thresholds. Stress, fear and a poor diet can all make a pain feel worse. A pain which worries you or is truly agonizing dominates your thinking and can prevent both mental and physical activities.

Swelling

Swelling is generally extra fluid which can form anywhere in the body as a result of injury, infection, disease, inflammation or disruption to the circulation. Fluid which forms as a result of injury is usually tissue fluid, blood, or synovial fluid, and is called fluid exudate. Blood in a joint is called a haemarthrosis. If blood forms an internal bruise it is a haematoma. An accumulation of tissue fluid is called oedema. When swelling consists of extra lymph fluid, it is known as lymphoedema. If the skin becomes dented when you press your finger into a swollen (oedematous) area, it is called pitting oedema.

Swelling gathers rapidly or slowly. It can look massive or slight on the surface. It can feel hot, cool, soft or firm to the touch. Swelling tends to track downwards under the influence of gravity, towards the foot from the leg, to the hand from the arm. This is called gravitational swelling.

When it appears in the early stages of an injury, swelling reflects the damage and inflammation. However, it can last beyond the healing stages. Chronic swelling can cause stiffness in the affected area, but is usually painless. It is a sign that the circulatory system has not yet recovered its efficiency and is not necessarily an indication that something is wrong.

If a painful hot swelling appears suddenly, especially in one or more joints, it can be a sign of an inflammatory condition such as rheumatoid arthritis (p. 12), infection (p. 13), or food intolerance (p. 11). This kind of swelling can occur out of the blue, or can coincide with an injury.

Complications

Injuries normally heal through natural processes. However, occasionally there are complications which delay healing. There may be hidden damage which was not obvious at the time of injury. Some complications are directly linked to the injury, including hidden organ damage, hidden tissue damage, non-healing, ischaemia, avascular necrosis and reflex sympathetic dystrophy. In other cases injuries are complicated by underlying conditions, such as food intolerance, circulatory problems, organ problems, inflammatory conditions and illnesses. Occasionally these conditions mimic injury pain, even when you have not hurt yourself.

Hidden organ damage

A direct blow or wound to the head or trunk carries the risk of damage to the organs, including the brain, spinal cord, spleen, kidneys, liver and heart.

Self-help for hidden organ damage
If there is any danger that you might have suffered internal damage or bleeding, you should be kept in hospital under observation for a suitable period of time, which is usually one to three days, depending on the circumstances.

Hidden tissue damage

Joint and soft tissue injuries such as a sprain or strain can be complicated by a subtle tear deep inside the tissues. Sometimes small slivers of bone or cartilage, known as 'loose bodies', form inside a joint. They usually cause a clicking sound when the joint moves, and occasionally block joint movement.

Joint damage can also lead to osteochondritis (osteochondrosis), or inflammation in the bone cartilage surfaces. If flakes of bone cartilage break off, the condition is called osteochondritis dissecans, which occurs particularly in the elbow and knee. If a ligament or tendon is badly strained near its attachment to a bone, a little bony outcrop – technically called an exostosis, spur or osteophyte – can appear at the edge of the bone. Small flakes of calcium can form in a soft tissue, causing irritation, and in a tendon this is termed calcific tendonitis. Following a muscle tear, bone fragments can form within the muscle tissue, causing pain and limitation of movement. This is myositis ossificans, and is most common in the front-thigh muscles (p. 122) and around the elbow (p. 282).

In children trauma can cause damage to the edges of the bones, rather than the soft tissues. Children often suffer avulsion fractures or epiphysis damage in situations which would cause ligament, tendon or muscle tears in an adult. Sometimes the diagnosis of bone damage is missed.

Self-help for hidden tissue damage
If your injury is not progressing as it should within a reasonable time frame, you should refer back to your practitioner in case there is damage which was missed at the time of your original assessment, or there is a problem which has arisen during the course of your recovery.

Non-healing

Broken bones sometimes fail to unite properly within a normal time frame. When a bone is slow to mend, the problem is termed 'delayed union'; when it fails altogether, it is 'non-union'. Non-union can happen in any broken bone, but is a particular risk if you break a bone with a poor blood supply, such as the talus in the ankle or the scaphoid in the wrist. Different factors contribute to delayed or non-healing, including mineral deficiency, infection and bone disease.

Self-help for non-healing
You should refer to your specialist for specific treatment and advice relevant to the cause of your problem. Generally, you should eat a healthy diet and avoid foods and drinks which might reduce body calcium. If in doubt, seek help from a professional nutritionist. If you smoke, you should stop, or at least cut down. You may need an operation to stabilize the fracture, treat an internal infection or stimulate bone growth.

Ischaemia

Sometimes an injury causes pressure on one or more arteries, leading to loss of blood flow in the injured area. An artery can be blocked or occluded by damage from broken or dislocated bone ends, and this is classified as Type I ischaemia. Type II ischaemia describes blood flow problems caused by internal bleeding or tissue swelling pressing on the artery, as in compartment syndrome, which can happen as an acute or overuse injury in the lower leg (p. 91) and the forearm (p. 278).

Interruption of the blood flow usually causes loss of the normal pulses and skin colour, and can result in severe pain, deformity, joint stiffness, muscle tightness and muscle shortening in the area normally supplied by the damaged arteries. When Type II ischaemia causes deformity and dysfunction in the arm or leg following an injury, the problem is known as Volkmann's ischaemic contracture.

Self-help for ischaemia
If you have suffered a traumatic injury which carries the risk of damaging the arteries, especially around the elbow, you should remain in hospital under observation for about 72 hours. If you develop the symptoms of arterial occlusion, you may need surgery by a vascular specialist to mend the damaged artery. If the ischaemia has been caused by compartment syndrome, you may need an operation called a fasciotomy to release the pressure which has blocked the blood flow.

Avascular necrosis

When a bone loses its blood supply, the substance of the bone can degenerate and bone cells die. The condition is called avascular necrosis or osteonecrosis, and it can follow bone fracture. It can affect any bone, including the talus in the ankle, the medial condyle of the femur at the knee, the head of the femur at the hip (p. 153), the top of the humerus at the shoulder, and the scaphoid in the wrist. Many different factors might contribute to the condition, including steroid use, alcoholism, circulatory problems like thrombosis, diabetes, certain medicines, some arthritic conditions including rheumatoid arthritis, and the pressure changes involved in deep-sea diving.

Self-help for avascular necrosis

If you develop a nagging deep pain with increasing stiffness following a bone fracture or dislocation, you should refer to your doctor or specialist. You may be sent for a magnetic resonance imaging (MRI) scan or possibly a bone scan, as X-rays usually look normal in the early stages of avascular necrosis. You should avoid painful activities, but you will probably be advised to do exercises to improve the blood supply to the affected area. Sometimes electrical stimulation is also used. The damaged bone might regenerate, but, if not, surgery may be recommended. You should take care of your diet, with help from a professional nutritionist or dietician if necessary. Avoid alcohol and smoking.

Reflex sympathetic dystrophy (RSD)

Reflex sympathetic dystrophy (RSD) is also known as causalgia, complex regional pain syndrome (CRPS) or Sudeck's atrophy. Its exact cause is not certain. RSD is a condition which can arise following apparently minor injuries. It can also follow operations, illnesses, including heart disease and breast cancer, and neurological conditions such as stroke or multiple sclerosis. It has been associated with taking barbiturates or drugs to treat tuberculosis.

RSD tends to occur mainly in the extremities. If it affects the foot, it can spread up the leg to the knee and even beyond. From the hand it can affect the elbow and then travel up to the shoulder. It can happen at any age, but is least common in very young children. It is more likely to happen in people who are anxious and tense, whether about their injury or generally. The condition is defined by its symptoms. The diagnosis is often missed in the early stages.

Symptoms of RSD

The affected area stops functioning normally. The skin over the affected area often turns a deep purplish-red colour, which is especially noticeable when you change position, for instance putting your foot to the floor as you get out of bed. At other times the skin may be unusually pale and shiny. It may feel clammy and sweaty, either hot to the touch, or abnormally cool. The skin hairs can disappear, or in some cases grow at an unusual rate.

Unusual, unexpected pain is characteristic. There is increased pain after or during even moderate exercise. The area becomes abnormally sensitive to the touch. Joints become tender and ever stiffer, while the muscles weaken, waste and tighten. If the condition develops, the bones in the area become thinner and weaker, and the nails of your fingers or toes may stop growing normally.

Treatments for RSD

Treatment is sometimes directed at the affected area, but this may aggravate the symptoms. The alternative is to activate the whole body, without emphasis on the painful part. For instance you can do exercises for the thigh and hip region when the foot is affected, or for the shoulder and upper arm if the problem is the hand. In all cases massage and acupuncture to the shoulder blade region can be helpful. Many RSD patients benefit from psychotherapy to alleviate underlying tension.

Individuals differ in their responses to the various treatments which might be offered for RSD. Some treatments are drastic, others more subtle. It takes time and patience to recover from RSD, and full recovery is always possible.

Self-help for RSD
- Look after your circulation (p. 27).
- Reduce stress.
- Practise relaxation techniques and deep-breathing exercises (p. 31).
- Keep your diet simple, and avoid irritants, especially caffeine and alcohol.
- Watch out for symptoms of food intolerance (p. 11).
- Find the right practitioner or team.
- If you are offered interventions like injections or surgery, make sure you are fully informed of the pros and cons.
- When you are confident you have found the right treatment or combination of treatments, follow the instructions to the letter.
- Always discuss with your practitioner(s) any fears or problems relating to the treatment.

Food intolerance

Food intolerance is an adverse reaction to foods, drinks, additives or preservatives. It is similar to allergy, but, unlike allergy, it is neither consistent nor constant.

Food intolerance can cause a wide variety of symptoms, including stiffness, swelling, heat and/or pain in one or more joints; muscular ache or cramping; nausea; vomiting; headache; skin blemishes; dry cracked skin, especially round the fingertips; irritability at the fingertips which makes you want to chew at the skin; eye soreness or dryness; and nose bleed. In children food intolerance is thought to be linked to hyperactivity. Gout can be considered a type of food intolerance.

Certain foodstuffs, artificial additives and preservatives are potential irritants. High-risk are caffeine, refined sugar and flour, dairy products, chocolates, acidic fruits like oranges and tomatoes, and spices. You can become intolerant to almost anything, including foods or drinks you are used to and which you consider healthy. Eating a lot of one type of food can lead to intolerance, for instance if you have a limited diet in which you eat and drink the same few things every day, or if you eat a lot of fruits such as plums or oranges because they are in season. Illness, infection, overtiredness and stress can make you more sensitive to potential irritants.

Self-help for food intolerance
- Keep a record of your food and drink intake and your symptoms.
- Eat regular, varied meals.
- Include plenty of fresh vegetables and non-irritant fruits in your diet.
- Eliminate any suspect foods or drinks.
- Avoid processed foods.
- Drink plain water regularly throughout the day.
- Avoid fruit juices and fizzy drinks.
- Avoid alcohol and caffeine.
- Do deep-breathing and relaxation exercises to reduce stress (p. 31).
- Rest and recover fully from any infection before resuming physical exercise.

Injuries and Diagnosis

Circulatory problems

Conditions, medicines and performance-enhancing drugs which affect the circulation can affect your muscles, especially in the calf and lower leg. You may get cramp-like feelings which seem like a muscle strain, even if you have done little or no exercise. There is tightness in the leg muscles, which makes you more vulnerable to injury when the muscles are stressed by activity.

Blood clots can form in the blood vessels for a variety of reasons. They are a risk factor following major injuries or complicated surgery, but can also happen in the leg veins if you sit still for too long, especially on a long-haul flight. When a blood clot forms in a vein there is usually a localized tender area, and a consistent sharp pain. The area may feel swollen, hardened and sometimes hot to the touch. A clot which forms in one of the deep-lying veins is called a deep vein thrombosis (DVT). If part of the clot breaks off, it is called an embolism. A pulmonary embolism is a clot which has lodged in the lungs, and is potentially fatal.

Self-help for circulatory problems
- Refer to your doctor or specialist as quickly as possible.
- Look after your circulation (p. 27).

Tip: Taking aspirin can help your arterial blood flow, but does not help to prevent venous blood clots.

Pain from the internal organs

Organs can transmit pain to the surface of the body: stomach problems can give rise to pain just under the left shoulder blade; spleen problems can cause pain in the left shoulder; inflammation of the diaphragm, liver abscess or gastric ulcer can cause pain over the right shoulder region; while the liver itself and the gall bladder can reflect pain just below the right shoulder blade. Heart conditions can cause pain round the left side of the chest to the sternum (breastbone), and down the left arm to the little finger.

Self-help for internal problems
- Make a note of all your symptoms.
- Rest.
- Alter your diet, if it seems relevant to the problem.
- Consult your doctor, who will refer you to an appropriate specialist for tests and treatment, if necessary.

Pain from inflammatory conditions

Inflammatory conditions like rheumatoid arthritis cause joint pain and swelling. In the early stages a sports player may not be aware of having a disease, and may confuse the symptoms with injury.

Self-help for inflammatory conditions
If you notice unexplained pain, swelling or other symptoms affecting your joints, try to work out what the cause might be. Seek specialist help through your doctor. Do not undertake heavy work or strenuous exercise. Changing your diet may make a difference to your symptoms. Simple measures may help, such as applying cold flannels or compresses with arnica or heparinoid cream (p. 29).

Pain caused by illness and infection

Pain can be caused or aggravated by viral and bacterial illnesses such as flu, glandular fever, meningitis and pleurisy. In many cases pain is felt around the neck, shoulder and chest regions, often accompanied by marked stiffness. Sometimes there is also aching or cramping in the calf muscles. The symptoms start unexpectedly, not always after physical activity. The pain and stiffness precede the symptoms of illness, such as a raised temperature, sore throat, swollen glands, cough or runny nose, which can appear as much as two weeks later.

More rarely, serious illnesses, including some cancerous tumours, can start with symptoms such as pain or swelling which mimic injury.

Bacterial infections which have been introduced through cuts in the skin or sexual contact can cause injury-like pain and swelling, especially in joints. You may have a raised temperature at the same time.

Gum disease not only causes toothache and pain in your mouth, but can also be linked to heart problems, stroke and females giving birth prematurely.

Ignoring the warning signs is dangerous. If you do strenuous exercise when you have an infection, you risk inflammation around or in the heart (pericarditis or myocarditis), or even sudden death.

Tips: Keep your anti-tetanus injections up to date. If you travel to areas of risk, make sure you have the recommended inoculations against diseases such as malaria. If you do water sports in polluted areas, carry written advice about Weil's disease (leptospirosis) to show to the casualty doctor, in case you are taken ill after falling in.

Self-help for illness or infection
- Stop or reduce all physical activities, especially if you have a raised temperature.
- Seek professional advice from your doctor or dentist, according to the symptoms.
- Rest lying down as much as possible during each day. Stay in bed if your symptoms are severe.
- Keep away from other people if you have an infectious illness.
- Never self-medicate with pharmaceutical, homeopathic or herbal remedies: always take professional advice.
- Do not do sport or demanding exercise while you are taking medicines, especially antibiotics.
- Allow several days after finishing a course of medicine so that your immune system regains strength before you take up sport again.
- Check your pulse first thing in the morning: if it is higher than normal and you feel tired or unwell, avoid strenuous exercise.
- Restart sport gradually and build up in easy stages.
- Allow rest phases in your daily schedule.
- Cut back physical activities immediately if you have signs of a recurrence of the illness or infection.

Pain from hormonal disturbances

Hormonal problems, changes due to the menstrual cycle and pregnancy, and taking medicines such as hormone replacement therapy (HRT) can make females more vulnerable to certain types of injury, as their ligaments tend to become lax, especially in the sacroiliac joints in the lower back. Some hormonal medicines, especially HRT, can themselves cause symptoms such as stiffness and pain in the muscles or joints.

Self-help for hormonal problems
- Keep a record of all your symptoms, activities, and food and fluid intake.
- Avoid rich or heavy foods, especially any which you feel a craving for.
- Make sure your diet is varied, with plenty of vegetables and fruit.
- Drink plain water regularly.
- Work out if any particular foods disagree with you.
- Seek professional help from your doctor or homeopath.

Diagnosis and assessment

An injury cannot be treated properly if there is uncertainty about what the damage is, and what has caused it. Investigations such as scans, X-rays or blood tests may be needed if your doctor or specialist feels that the injury may be serious enough to need surgery or if it is possible that your problem is caused or complicated by an illness or inflammatory condition. Investigations are not infallible. X-rays, for instance, usually fail to show up a stress fracture in the early stage. When operating, surgeons often find unexpected defects which were not evident on scans beforehand.

Tip: Avoid unnecessary investigations. X-rays and CT scans in particular involve high levels of radiation.

Diagnosis in sports injuries is based on the description of what has happened (technically known as the history) and the physical assessment. It is not something you can do for yourself unless you have appropriate professional training. The sports injury practitioner has to have a sound knowledge of anatomy, biomechanics, injuries and injury mechanisms, treatment options, contra-indications and possible complications, as well as an awareness of the problems and diseases which can masquerade as sports injuries or which might be present alongside an injury.

Self-help for diagnosis

The history is all-important. To help your practitioner make the right diagnosis, you should keep a written record of what happened and as many background factors as you can. In the case of a child, either a parent or a responsible adult should piece the story together.

Guidelines for your record:

Your injury and symptoms
- When and how did your injury happen or your pain start?
- What was the pain like then?

- Did you have other symptoms, such as an open wound, swelling, stiffness, numbness, skin colour changes, instability, catching, locking, clicking or grinding?
- Did you have any kind of infection around the time of the injury?
- Have you noticed any other symptoms such as headache, stomach upset, or joint or muscle aches?
- What is the pain like now, and what brings it on?
- Can you relieve your pain and symptoms? If so, how?
- Have you had any treatment for the problem? If so, what was the treatment and was it helpful?
- Can you still do your sport?
- Does your injury interfere with your normal life?

Previous problems
- Have you had any previous injuries or problems in the same area? If so, when?
- Have you had any other injuries or accidents in the past?
- (teenagers and adults) Did you suffer from 'growing pains' as a young child?
- Have you ever had any significant illnesses, such as glandular fever, meningitis, hepatitis, rheumatic fever, bronchitis or pneumonia?

General health
- Do you have any health problems, such as asthma, diabetes, high cholesterol or blood pressure?
- Do you tend to get cramp, particularly in the legs, at night or other times?
- Do you tend to get breathless or suffer from headaches?
- Do you have any problems with your teeth and gums?
- Do you suffer from any allergies?
- Are your bowel movements normal and regular?
- Is your urine a normal light yellowish colour, and do you pass urine regularly without difficulty or urgency?
- (females) Is your menstrual cycle regular and normal?
- (females) Are you, or might you be pregnant?
- (females) Do you take any medicines such as the contraceptive pill or HRT?

Lifestyle
- What is your job, or your main activity each day?
- What do you like doing for recreation?
- Do you participate in sport and/or exercise regularly?
- Are you in training for a particular sport? If so, what kind of training do you do?
- Do you eat regular meals, including vegetables and fruit?
- How much plain water do you drink each day?
- Do you take any supplements, whether vitamins, minerals or performance-enhancing drugs?
- Do you smoke? If so, how much each day?
- Do you drink alcohol, if so how much and how often?
- Do you suffer from anxiety, overtiredness or stress?

Injuries and Diagnosis

The right practitioner

Different injuries require different treatments and therefore different practitioners. Sometimes a team is needed to deal with the different factors involved in an injury. Finding the right practitioner(s) or clinic is not always straightforward, even if you opt to pay for your treatment privately. If you have medical insurance, you have to comply with the conditions in order to make a claim.

In most developed countries your family doctor has to refer you to specialists for treatment, although you may be able to see a complementary practitioner – such as a physical therapist / physiotherapist, athletic trainer, osteopath, chiropractor, podiatrist, nutritionist or dietician – without a referral. 'Alternative' complementary practitioners – such as homeopaths, acupuncturists, reflexologists, masseurs, shiatsu and Bowen practitioners and applied kinesiologists – can usually be consulted directly. Ethical practitioners from any profession may offer to keep your doctor informed of their part in your treatment, whether or not there was a referral.

If your injury requires an operation, make sure you are informed of what the operation entails, and any possible risks. Try to find the best specialist for your problem. Many orthopaedic surgeons specialize in a particular part of the body or a certain type of surgery. In some countries, notably the United States, podiatrists are not only specialists in foot biomechanics and the prescription of custom-made orthotics, but also qualified to do foot surgery. You are entitled to ask about the surgeon's experience and success rate with the particular procedure, and whether the consultant surgeon would do the operation personally, or give responsibility for it to a more junior assistant. If in doubt, ask your doctor to refer you for a second specialist opinion.

Tips:
- *Be suitably dressed for your consultation. Shorts and T-shirt or modest underwear are called for in case you are asked to undress.*
- *Give your doctor or practitioner full information about your problem at every stage.*
- *Only consult practitioners who have relevant qualifications and experience.*
- *Never consult different practitioners without reference to each other.*
- *Ask your practitioner to explain your diagnosis and treatment.*
- *Follow your chosen practitioner's instructions faithfully.*
- *Tell your practitioner if you have any doubts about the treatment methods, or any adverse reactions.*
- *If you feel treatment is not working, seek a second opinion through your doctor.*
- *Allow time for the injury to heal completely and for the rehabilitation programme to have its effect.*
- *Be positive, patient and flexible: accept any setbacks, and keep working towards recovery.*

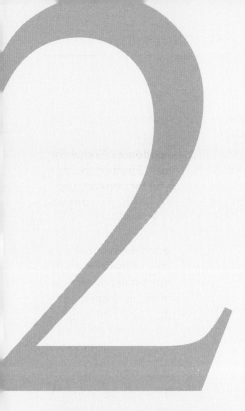

Rehabilitation Explained

Every injury impairs function to some degree. Most kinds of tissue damage will heal naturally, but that is only part of your recovery. You also have to retrain the muscles and nerves in the damaged area, to recover normal patterns of coordination. An accurate and detailed rehabilitation exercise programme is an essential part of injury treatment. This applies to children's injuries just as much as adults'. Functional recovery is the aim of rehabilitation.

Nature blocks movement around an injured area in order to prevent further damage and allow healing. There may be pain, stiffness, muscle spasm, swelling or actual obstruction by damaged or displaced structures. Most important is the loss of coordination caused by disturbance in the nerve systems. 'Proprioception' and 'kinaesthetic sense' are terms meaning your in-built awareness of the different parts of your body, which is vital for balance and coordinated movement.

Healing depends on the right kind of exercise in each phase. Even in the earliest stages of a major injury, you should be doing activities to promote recovery and prevent secondary damage and circulatory complications such as blood clots (p. 12). Active rehabilitation starts as soon as the acute phase of your injury is over. The timing varies according to the nature and severity of the injury. After an operation, or if your problem is complicated, your surgeon, doctor or specialist will tell you when you can and should start to do remedial exercises. The remedial programme is usually the responsibility of a rehabilitation practitioner, most often a physical therapist / physiotherapist or athletic trainer. For foot-related problems, a podiatrist or chiropodist may be involved.

The majority of sports injuries are musculoskeletal problems involving the bones and soft tissues, and they are treated by practitioners with musculoskeletal or orthopaedic training and experience. For the rarer cases involving the central nervous system, with brain or spinal cord damage, treatment is best done by specialist neurological therapists.

For many sports injuries the rehabilitation practitioner is responsible for treatment from day one. You should wear sports kit for your sessions. Skilful rehabilitation consists of several elements:

- assessing which movements or activities are blocked or impaired;
- analysing why normal movements are no longer possible;
- setting realistic goals;
- giving treatments which create the conditions for functional recovery;
- setting out and supervising the remedial exercise programme;
- constructing a fitness programme to maintain and improve overall condition;
- recognising and correcting setbacks;
- preventing future injuries.

Assessing movement impairment

The rehabilitation practitioner watches how you hold yourself, move about, and what position you take up when you sit or lie down, noting which movements are difficult or impossible, which you can do by using compensatory movements, and which are unaffected.

Your movements can be tested passively and actively. For passive tests you relax completely, and the practitioner checks how well your joints and their component parts move and how pliable your soft tissues are. For active testing, the practitioner asks you to perform certain movements, giving you some support or help if necessary. To test muscles and tendons, the practitioner may resist the movement. The positions chosen for these tests must be safe and comfortable. You might stand up, sit on a chair, or lie on a treatment couch on your back, stomach or side.

Patterns of movement are tested by the practitioner using subtle hand pressures to guide you as you activate the movements. This shows whether your coordinated actions in any direction have been affected by your injury. The movements can involve complex patterns of rotation, combined with flexion or extension in any part of the body. They can be the basis for active manual treatments (p. 21). This type of testing is often used for musculoskeletal injuries, but especially for cases where there is neurological damage from a head or spinal injury.

Analysing the causes of movement impairment

Movement impairment can be caused by tissue damage, such as a broken bone or torn tendon; mechanical block, such as loose bodies in a joint; pain; swelling; muscle inhibition; muscle spasm; nerve disruption; or a combination of these factors. In neurological damage there may be spasticity (uncontrollable muscle tightening or hypertonia) or flaccidity (hypotonia) coupled with overcompensation mechanisms. Sometimes a disease or inflammatory condition (p. 12) causes symptoms which seem like an injury. Your description of your problem (p. 14) is vital, and the rehabilitation practitioner also has to watch for the signs distinguishing injury from other problems.

Setting realistic goals

From the initial physical assessment, goals are set within the recovery programme.

Timescales vary according to the injury. Each patient is individual, and some recover more quickly than others. The rehabilitation practitioner has to allow for this, and develop the recovery programme at the rate which suits you. It is very disappointing if you have been told that you should be running or playing your sport within a certain time and it does not happen. Positive thinking plays an important part in recovery, but trying too hard can hold you back. Deadlines can be dangerous. Professional sports players are often pushed back into competition in the shortest possible time – usually shorter than possible. Too often they pay the price with re-injury, secondary injuries or prematurely arthritic joints.

Functional recovery takes longer than tissue healing. For instance, a torn Achilles tendon can knit together naturally within two to four weeks, but it takes several months to strengthen up. Similarly, a broken weight-bearing bone needs a year or more to recover fully, although it will normally mend itself within a few weeks. It takes about three months for muscles to adapt to a training programme for improving flexibility and strength, but much longer if the nerve systems have been impaired.

The aim of rehabilitation is your return to all the sports and activities you enjoy and wish to do. However, certain injuries can put you out of your sport, especially if you are a professional or elite sports competitor and suffer an injury late in your career. Any major injury at any age is likely to mean the end of sports like gymnastics, American football, rugby, show jumping and rock climbing, but it may be possible to do other types of sport. Injuries involving the central nervous system, with damage to the brain or spinal cord, can leave you partially disabled or confined to a wheelchair, although full recovery is not impossible. For wheelchair users, there is a wide range of sports. The Paralympics have grown in size and status, offering opportunities for high-level competition to those who enjoy that motivation.

In all cases, you should progress through your rehabilitation programme step by step until you are fully fit.

Rehabilitation treatment

There are many physical treatments which help reduce pain and swelling, release tightness and promote tissue healing. These include manual therapy such as massage and manipulation, and electrotherapy, for instance laser, interferential and ultrasound. For functional recovery you have to be active. Rehabilitation practitioners set exercise programmes. Many use active neuromuscular training techniques, including electrical muscle stimulation to help you exercise more effectively.

Treatment sessions are given according to the injury and the needs of the patient. While a professional or elite sports competitor might be treated several times a day, a recreational player may be treated just once a week or once a fortnight. For many common injuries, treatment as such is not needed, if the patient can be advised at intervals on what to do. In all cases the patient has to take a certain level of responsibility for the recovery process, and work at the remedial programme.

Electrical muscle stimulation

Neuromuscular electrical stimulation, or electrical muscle stimulation (EMS), is an effective method for retraining nerve-muscle action. Injuries cause inhibition of the muscles in the injured area, whether or not the muscles themselves have been damaged. EMS helps to restore precise muscle action, and to prevent compensatory movements. For the main fast-twitch motor muscles (p. 22), the stimulation is usually done using a rate of 40–50 hertz (pulses per second, or pps), which is close to the natural frequency at which a motor nerve fires. This type of stimulation works only if the muscle has a working motor nerve, not if it is denervated. When the motor nerve is inhibited, it can take up to 80 milliamperes (mA) or more to activate it, whereas a healthy motor nerve reacts at about 18–20 mA. Stimulating the nerve makes an innervated muscle contract, but this does not increase strength by itself. You have to work with the current and actively contract the muscle in order to improve efficiency in the nerve-muscle coordination, which is the basis for improving strength.

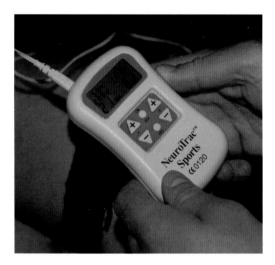

A compact electrical muscle stimulator.

For slow-twitch postural muscles (p. 22) a low frequency is used – usually 10–15 pps. This can increase muscle efficiency without you having to contract the muscles actively. It can be useful for conditions such as compartment syndrome (p. 91), or in situations where the muscles have been weakened by damage to the nervous system. It has a strong effect on the circulation, so it is applied gradually, starting with very short periods, to avoid unwanted side effects such as headaches.

EMS can also be a home treatment, once you have been shown exactly how to use it safely.

Manual therapy

Through hand contact the practitioner can feel the state of the patient's tissues in and around the injured area, as well as any reactions to the techniques being applied. Manual therapy is individual, and is constantly developing as practitioners modify or add to the basic methods they learned during their training. Most manual therapists enhance their skills by learning from practitioners in a wide variety of complementary professions.

Passive techniques
Some treatments, generally based on massage or manipulation, are applied by the practitioner without you having to do anything. Soft tissue release can be used to ease tight tissues, reduce spasm and improve the localized blood flow. Some of the many techniques for doing this are subtle, others more forceful. Passive movements are a simple technique to keep joints moving, improve the circulatory flow and prevent stiffness when you cannot move the joints for yourself. Joint manipulations are a more complex form of passive movements, and range from very gentle to full-thrust. There are also systems in which gentle, subtle energy is applied to your tissues to stimulate healing responses, including craniosacral therapy and the Bowen technique.

Activating treatments

There are many systems of guided or resisted exercises, in which you participate as the practitioner leads the movements. The practitioner chooses precise patterns of movements, and can feel when a movement is difficult for you, or when you start to use compensatory actions.

This type of exercise uses your proprioceptive feedback mechanisms: the practitioner's hands give your nerve-muscle system a signal to respond to, creating a challenge so that your responses become more efficient. Sometimes the practitioner gives you verbal instructions, sometimes not. Movements may be guided, so that you activate your muscles to follow as the practitioner's hands lead in a certain direction, or resisted, with the practitioner blocking your movement to make you contract the muscles as hard as you can without pain or inhibition. The practitioner controls the exact amount of work you have to do so that it is difficult, but always possible.

These manual therapies include proprioceptive neuromuscular facilitation (PNF), muscle energy techniques (METs), shiatsu, neuromuscular energizing therapy (NET) and many others which have been developed by individual therapists according to similar or parallel principles.

The remedial exercise programme

After a bone injury, you have to re-strengthen all the muscles in the area, retrain soft tissue flexibility and joint mobility, and allow time for the bone itself to strengthen. For any joint injury, you have to recover stability round the joint by strengthening the muscles and tendons, and then work on improving mobility while continuing to work on strengthening exercises. For an injured muscle, you need to work on regaining flexibility and strength through the muscle's range of movement. An injured tendon requires stability and re-strengthening combined with gentle flexibility work.

If you have been in bed following an operation, the priority is to strengthen your weakened muscles and help you to get up, so that you can get out of bed independently and safely. You may need to use crutches for walking in the early stages of recovery (p. 32).

Every remedial exercise has a precise purpose, so it has to be constructed and performed accurately. Each has a starting position and an action. It can be performed against gravity, in the direction of gravity, against resistance, or with assistance. The purpose can be to strengthen or stretch muscle, increase joint mobility, or improve neuromuscular coordination and proprioception. Attention to detail is vital.

The programme gradually builds up. Progression involves increasing the repetitions and sets of each exercise, and then increasing the difficulty, for instance by adding weight resistance or including more complex exercises. As you regain function in the injured area, activities related to your sport can be included in the programme, but you must recover fully before resuming your normal training and playing routines.

Exercises explained

Muscles

Voluntary muscles are those you use for actions. Normal muscle is always in a state of slight tension called 'muscle tone', which varies according to the individual. A fit, energetic person tends to have high tone, whereas muscles may be low tone in someone who is untrained or depressed. Following major damage to the central nervous system, tone can be abnormally high ('spastic') or low ('flaccid').

Active muscles are divided into two main groups: fast-twitch and slow-twitch. Those consisting mainly of fast-twitch fibres contract at speed, and tend to lie nearer the surface of the body, such as gastrocnemius (p. 71). Slow-twitch muscles, such as soleus (p. 71), lie more deeply, closer to the bones. They have a richer blood supply, tire less easily, and work consistently to keep you upright against the effect of gravity. All muscle activity is triggered by nerve impulses.

Muscles which perform an action are known as 'agonists' or 'prime movers', while the opposite muscle groups or 'antagonists' have to pay out: this is called 'reciprocal action'. For instance, biceps brachii contracts as triceps lengthens and relaxes when you bend your elbow against gravity or a resistance. Muscles which collaborate in a movement, usually by providing stability, are known as 'synergists'. For example, the rotator cuff tendons steady the humerus when you lift your arm up.

Remedial exercises

Remedial dynamic exercises can be classified as non-weight-bearing (NWB), partial weight-bearing (PWB) or full weight-bearing (FWB). After a leg injury, you may have to keep your body weight off the leg at first, progressing in stages until you can take full weight. Arm movements such as lifting sideways from the shoulder into abduction are non-weight-bearing, press-ups are partial weight-bearing and handstands are full weight-bearing.

Exercises can also be defined as open kinetic chain (OKC) and closed kinetic chain (CKC). In OKC exercises a limb is moved freely in the air, as in a straight-leg raise (p. 115), or arm abduction (p. 258). In CKC exercises the movement is done with the end of the limb fixed, for instance the hip raise in crook-lying (p. 162), standing squats (p. 128) and press-ups (p. 311).

Starting positions

The starting position provides the basis for every exercise. For early stage remedial exercises the starting position provides support for performing simple movements, and is stable enough to prevent unwanted movements. In later stages the base of support is reduced to provide more of a challenge. The most stable base of support is lying flat, whether on your stomach or your back, while the least stable is standing on tiptoe on one leg, especially on a soft or mobile surface.

Strengthening exercises

Strengthening exercises are dynamic or static.

Dynamic exercises

Working dynamically, you perform a movement against gravity or using a resistance such as your body weight, pulleys, springs, exercise bands, dumb-bells, free weights or fixed-weights machines. When your muscles work against gravity or a load, they shorten, and this is called 'concentric work'. On the return movement, working in the opposite direction under the influence of gravity or the load, the muscles pay out and lengthen as they control the movement: this is called 'eccentric work', and is a vital part of rehabilitation. If you do several repetitions of a dynamic exercise quickly, you add aerobic training to the strengthening action. To gain strength you have to increase the difficulty of each exercise in stages, for instance by adding to the weight resistance, doing the exercise more quickly, or increasing the repetitions or sets.

Tip: When you do dynamic strength exercises, only increase the workload or resistance in gradual, manageable stages.

Exercise machines

Most fixed-weights machines provide concentric and eccentric training for the working muscles, whereas machines using hydraulic resistance provide concentric training for opposing muscle groups. Isokinetic machines offer sophisticated strength exercises and measurements, in which the resistance adapts to the amount of force you apply through the movement, and your strength through the range can be analysed instantly.

Range of movement

The major moving joints in the body have a range of movement, creating an arc from the close-packed position in the inner range, through the middle range, extending to a fully stretched position in the outer range. Dynamic exercises are done using part or all of the range in a joint. You can apply maximum strength in the middle range, and this is how bodybuilders train to increase muscle bulk. However, for functional strength relevant to both sport and injury prevention you need strength through the whole range, so most dynamic rehabilitation and conditioning exercises go from a pre-stretch to the close-packed position whenever possible.

Isometric exercises

Static or isometric muscle work entails applying your effort against an unmoving resistance to increase muscle tension. This can be done at any point in a joint's range of movement. You normally hold the contraction for about three to five seconds, and then relax completely to let the blood flow freely again. Isometric exercise can be invaluable in the early stages following any injury, and later on if there are specific points of weakness in a muscle group. It is used specifically to correct overmobile hyperextending elbow (p. 272) or knee (p. 100) joints.

Caution: Isometric training has a strong effect on the circulation, and can increase your blood pressure, so it is not recommended for people with any kind of heart or circulatory problem, unless under direct medical supervision.

Rehabilitation Explained

Stretching and mobilizing

Stretching and mobilizing exercises are done to prevent stiffness and to increase the pliability of your body. They help your circulation and are an important part of body conditioning training, both for sport and for health. Injury causes tissue tightness, partly as a protective mechanism and partly through inhibition because of pain. Loosening the injured area is an important part of the recovery process.

What stretching does
Stretching improves elasticity in your muscles, skin and fasciae (the connective tissues which surround the major structures of the body and divide the body into compartments), and to a lesser extent in the stiffer soft tissues such as tendons and ligaments.

How to stretch
The safe way to stretch a muscle group is to contract the opposite muscles as much as you comfortably can, placing the muscles at their full natural length, and then push or pull the limb just a little further. For instance, to stretch the front-thigh muscles, lie on your front, bend one knee, then pull the ankle gently towards your bottom (p. 126). Hold the stretched position still for a count of six, breathing evenly, then relax completely.

When to stretch
This type of stretching is safe when the muscles are cold, first thing in the morning or before your warm-up, as you are stretching within the muscles' elastic limits. If a muscle group is specially tight, perhaps after heavy training, you should stretch patiently until it is fully flexible again before putting it under strain. Passive stretching at the end of a hard exercise session can help prevent after-stiffness.

Which muscles?
Stretching the major muscle groups of the arms and legs is relatively straightforward, as they are arranged more or less in lines. Overstretching must be avoided, as it can cause damage. Do not hold the stretch for too long. You should never force the stretch, nor push further into a stretch from the stretched position. If you do, the muscles may appear to have stretched out considerably at the time, but will then quickly revert to their original tightness. You have to take special care when trying to stretch the spinal muscles, because the complex arrangement of short and long muscles means it is all too easy to pull too hard and cause damage to the little muscles or ligaments.

Mobilizing exercises
Mobilizing exercises loosen joints and improve local blood flow. They are rhythmic ballistic bouncing movements, done gently, without any major effort. Examples include arm circling and gentle trunk twisting, side bending or flexion-extension movements.

Alternative fitness training

Through all the recovery phases, alternative fitness work is done to maintain and improve your overall body balance and condition. The better you maintain your general fitness, the easier it is to return safely to sport. If in the past you have only been doing your sport without background fitness and conditioning training, you will be better off after a rehabilitation programme which includes these elements.

The type and amount of alternative training you can do depends on your injury. The programme should include strengthening and flexibility exercises for all the parts of your body which are not affected by your injury, and cardiovascular or aerobic exercise for your heart and lungs. A moderately strenuous workout lasting about 20–30 minutes twice a week will maintain or even improve your general fitness.

The professional or elite sports player needs to be active every day, as much for psychological as physical reasons, so the programme has to be varied. The basis can be a combination of endurance and speed work, using circuit exercises for speed and local muscle endurance, and longer spells of steady-state exercise for overall endurance.

Choosing training activities

If you have a leg injury, you can achieve a worthwhile level of aerobic work for the heart and lungs by exercising your arms. A leg injury invariably means you cannot run, but you may be able to do other types of exercise using the injured leg. For example, with a ruptured Achilles tendon (p. 76), you may be able to work out on an exercise bike in the protective cast, using your heel. A removable boot allows you to shower or take a bath normally. If you have a plaster cast, you have to wrap it carefully in a plastic covering before showering.

With certain injuries, especially in the later stages, you may be able to exercise in a pool, combining remedial exercises for your injury with swimming, general exercises, walking or even running in the water. Activities such as yoga and Pilates may also be possible.

Sport-related activities

It may be possible to incorporate modified activities related to your sport in the alternative fitness programme. If your sport is one-sided, it is very helpful if you can do simulated movements using the non-dominant side, such as shadow strokes for tennis or golf, or throwing actions for baseball, javelin or shot putting. After recovery, using the non-dominant side in this way can be helpful in preventing re-injury.

New skills

An injury which prevents you from doing your own sport can be an opportunity to try out a different activity and learn new skills. An injured footballer or runner might discover archery, canoeing or golf, for instance, or an injured tennis player can get interested in rowing or weightlifting. These new experiences contribute to the player's physical and psychological wellbeing.

Rehabilitation Explained

Setbacks

Sometimes things go wrong in a recovery programme, or appear to; your progress stalls, or you may even retrogress. Possible reasons are:

- you have not followed instructions properly;
- you have done your exercises incorrectly;
- you have been impatient and tried to do too much;
- you have done too little;
- you have consulted various practitioners and tried to mix different lines of treatment;
- the original diagnosis was incorrect, or the assessment inadequate;
- your practitioner has set inappropriate exercises;
- your practitioner has set the programme incorrectly;
- your practitioner has failed to monitor your exercises closely enough;
- your practitioner has tried to push you too hard.

Whatever the cause, the situation can usually be rectified. You and your practitioner must check out why you are no longer making progress, and adapt your programme accordingly. You may decide to seek advice from a different rehabilitation practitioner. If there is doubt about the original diagnosis, you need to refer back to your doctor or specialist, or seek a second opinion.

Injury prevention

You need to understand how your injury happened in order to prevent it from recurring or leading to further injuries. Your practitioner should explain the relevant factors to you. Your rehabilitation and alternative fitness programmes can form the basis of injury prevention exercises ('prehab'), which you should do regularly, even after you have recovered.

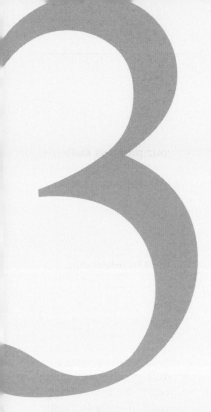

Chapter 3

Injuries and Self-Help

There is no point trying to play through or 'run off' an injury. Any activity which causes pain, whether during or afterwards, must be avoided. There are simple measures you can take to help healing and relieve your symptoms when an injury happens. Never take risks. If there are any signs of increased pain, seek professional help as soon as possible.

Circulatory care

Good blood flow is an important part of general health, and is vital for promoting healing and preventing complications after an injury or operation. You need to prevent congestion in the circulatory system, and to promote the action of the heart, lungs and blood vessels. Many different internal and external factors are involved.

1. Drink plain water

- make plain water the main part of your fluid intake;
- drink water little and often at regular intervals throughout the day, starting from first thing in the morning;
- do not wait until you are thirsty before drinking;
- drink before, during and after exercise;
- drink more if you are in a hot or humid climate;
- if you find it difficult to drink normal water, filter or heat it before drinking;
- avoid using plastic bottles;
- avoid or limit caffeinated, alcoholic, fizzy and sweet drinks.

2. Eat a healthy diet

- eat regular meals, including vegetables and fruits;
- avoid processed and 'junk' foods;
- make sure you take in enough salt, but not too much, to maintain adequate mineral levels;
- consult your doctor or a dietician or nutritionist for professional advice.

Tip: Do not take any over-the-counter herbal or pharmaceutical medicines for your circulation, except with guidance from your practitioner.

3. Bed rest and circulatory care

If you have had a bad accident or a major operation, you may have to stay in bed for a period of time. You should keep the unaffected parts of your body moving, doing exercises at least every hour. Your practitioner may suggest some of the following:

- do deep-breathing exercises;
- circle your feet and move them up and down at the ankles;
- tighten your thigh muscles to straighten your knees as hard as you can;
- bend, straighten and lift each knee in turn;
- lift your arms upwards and reach above your head;
- bend and straighten your elbows;
- exercise your hands and fingers;
- tighten and relax your stomach muscles;
- move your head gently in all directions;
- change position if you can, to lie on your stomach or each side.

4. Use slings and supports correctly

Immobilization is used for major injuries such as bone fracture, joint dislocation and tendon rupture, and for more minor problems like tenosynovitis. It is not used where movement is important for healing, for instance in stress fractures, except to prevent the patient from doing harmful activities. When it is necessary to limit movement and control swelling, a hinged brace or padded bandaging can be used for the arm or leg. An adjustable brace is used when range of movement has to be increased by stages, for instance following Achilles tendon rupture (p. 76) or some types of knee problem. To support the back or neck, you may use a flexible or rigid corset or collar (brace).

Supports or bandages should always cover an area beyond the actual injury on an arm or leg, to avoid impeding the blood flow. Once a support has been fitted, you must watch for warning signs such as skin irritation, increased pain, or your toes or fingers turning white, blue, numb and/or cold below the splint. If necessary, refer back to your practitioner urgently so that the support can be removed or adjusted.

Tip: Do not use a tight sleeve- or stocking-type support on your leg or arm for any length of time as it may restrict blood flow and hinder nerves.

When an injury has caused long-term weakness and instability, as in 'weak ankles' (p. 62) or after cruciate ligament rupture (p. 102), you may be advised to use a splint or support indefinitely, especially for sports. There are many types of support available over-the-counter, but it is best to be guided by your practitioner.

Tips: Do not use a support or taping in order to continue doing activities which would otherwise cause pain. Do not try to drive if you cannot do an emergency stop, or if you have to use a neck brace, as your insurance is invalid.

5. Use hot and cold treatments

Ice and cold compresses can help reduce swelling and control pain. There are various ways of applying ice. I recommend simple ice massage: gently pass an ice cube over the injured area for five to ten seconds, dab the skin dry, then repeat three or four times, until the skin has reddened slightly. The aim is to stimulate the circulation and prevent secondary damage.

Contrast baths have the same purpose. Fill two basins or buckets, one with water which is comfortably hot, not boiling, and the other with cold water and some ice cubes. Dip the injured area into one bucket for a few seconds, dab it dry, then into the other bucket, and repeat a few times until the skin has reddened slightly.

Do not leave ice or an ice pack on the skin for so long that the area becomes white and numb. You risk burning the skin and slowing down healing by suppressing the blood flow and reducing the normal inflammatory response to injury.

Cold treatments and contrast baths are mainly used as first-aid treatments, but they can also be used in the later stages of an injury, for example if you have persistent gravitational swelling in a joint (p. 7).

A warm bath or shower can also help to stimulate the circulation and relieve pain.

6. How to use creams, liniments, oils and ointments

For many injuries you can use a cream or ointment to help the circulation and soothe discomfort. There are many types of ointment and lotion which claim to help injuries. Always look at the ingredients and formulation, be guided by your practitioner, and only buy reputable brands.

Tip: Heat-producing creams or liniments are not suitable for the early stages of an injury, as they might cause congestion in the tissues.

Most relevant to injuries, especially in the early stages, are heparinoid creams or gels (pharmaceutical products specifically for the circulation, which are sold under various brand names) or the herbal remedies arnica or St. John's wort oil.

You should not rub an injured area hard, especially in the early stages. Cream or ointment should be applied lightly at the edges of the injured area, if it is very sore or if there is an open wound. For a joint injury which is causing swelling, you can use poultices (compresses) directly over the swelling to help the circulation and control the exudate: put your lotion, ointment or cream on one or more gauze swabs, depending on the area to be covered; place the swab over the swollen area, or a swab on either side of the joint, and fix it in place with a crepe bandage which extends well above and below the level of the injury.

Watch out for any signs of discomfort, allergy or infection. If they occur, remove the dressings straight away, wash the area with water and refer to your practitioner.

7. Use tablets and supplements with care

It used to be the norm for doctors to recommend tablets, especially anti-inflammatories, for injuries, but later research showed that these medicines might suppress the normal inflammatory reaction which is part of tissue healing. Many medicines have side effects, so if you choose to take them, always read the instructions and follow your doctor's advice.

Vitamin and mineral supplements may be needed for certain problems, for instance if you have any degree of iron deficiency. Your practitioner might also recommend supplements to help healing, such as glucosamine for joint problems, or vitamin C for wounds or muscle and tendon injuries. If you take supplements, keep to the recommended dose. Stop taking them and refer back to your practitioner if you feel any adverse reactions.

Always seek medical guidance if you wish to take performance-enhancing supplements or drugs. Most have side-effects: for example, steroids can weaken your bones and tendons, and can have even more serious consequences, especially if taken long-term.

Do not self-medicate. Keep all your practitioners informed of any medicines or supplements you are taking. Remember that supplements and medicines alone cannot cure an injury problem. A rehabilitation programme is always essential for full functional recovery.

Tip: Do not take painkilling tablets in order to do activities which would otherwise be painful.

8. Avoid direct pressure or constriction

- do not cross your legs or ankles when sitting or lying down;
- do not wear tight shoes or clothing;
- wear flexible shoes with a low heel;
- use cushioning insoles or heel pads in your shoes;
- do not sit or lie still on hard surfaces for any length of time.

9. Keep good posture

- sit and stand straight and symmetrically;
- avoid sitting or standing still for long periods;
- move about as much as you can;

- use a rocking chair for relaxation;
- avoid lounging or curling up on a sofa;
- sit at a table to read or to use your computer or laptop;
- arrange your desk height so that your hands are at a comfortable level for writing or using a keyboard;
- place your computer screen high enough so that you look straight at it, not downwards.

10. Prevent gravitational swelling

- when sitting or lying down, put your legs up on a soft support so that your feet are above the level of your hips;
- to control leg swelling, lift the foot of your bed up on to blocks about ten centimetres (four inches) high. If you have high blood pressure, ask for your doctor's advice before doing this;
- use Chinese iron balls to exercise your hand and stimulate the circulation: rotate them round the palm using your fingers and thumb, trying not to let the two spheres touch each other;
- place a golf ball or foot massager on the floor and rub your foot over it for a few minutes at a time;
- use support stockings or bandaging for leg swelling, or a sling for the arm if your practitioner has recommended you should.

11. De-stress

Even ten minutes a day spent relaxing or meditating can have a significant effect on your blood pressure. You can learn relaxation techniques in a class or individually, or try some of the following simple methods:

- working from the feet upwards, think of each part of your body in turn, tense the muscles two or three times, then release them;
- imagine yourself floating in a calm lagoon;
- imagine your whole body being pleasantly bathed in your favourite colour, or any beautiful colour that comes to mind;
- think of yourself resting or doing a favourite activity in a beautiful place;
- if negative or stressful thoughts intrude, take a few deep breaths and imagine them floating away and disappearing each time you breathe out.

12. Breathe deeply

Deep breathing has a beneficial effect on the heart and lungs, and helps to reduce tension. You can learn deep-breathing techniques from a variety of practitioners, or try this simple method: sit or lie down comfortably, breathe in deeply through your nose, expanding your ribcage, then breathe out through your mouth, feeling your ribs sink down and in so that you expel the air completely; do three to four deep breaths at a time, then rest. You can repeat this about five times whenever you choose.

Tip: Avoid being in a smoky atmosphere. If you smoke, try to stop, or at least cut down.

Injuries and Self-Help

Getting back on your feet using crutches

When you cannot walk properly due to a foot or leg problem, a walking aid allows you to get around without making your injury worse, and helps to prevent secondary problems caused by limping. In some cases you might need a walking frame, but more often crutches are used.

There are two types of crutches. Elbow crutches, usually made of metal, are lightweight and relatively easy to use. Axillary crutches, which may be wooden or metal, are more cumbersome, but are considered safer for heavy patients.

Crutches have to be the right height. The handles should feel comfortable, and may need padding if they are hard. The rubber tips under the crutches, called ferrules, are vital for preventing slipping. If they get lost or worn down, they must be replaced immediately.

Adjusting crutches for height

Wearing shoes, stand up straight with your arms by your sides, with the crutches beside you, not in your hands. The handles of the crutches should be level with the ulnar head on either side, the bone which juts out just above the little finger side of your wrist.

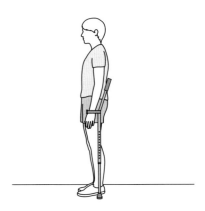

For axillary crutches, the tops of the crutches should rest about eight centimetres (three inches) below the armpits, or about two-thirds up the arm between the elbow and the shoulder. Otherwise pressure from the crutches against your armpits can damage the nerves and cause discomfort or even temporary paralysis down to your hands.

Walking with crutches

Crutches are used to keep weight off your injured leg, either totally in non-weight-bearing mode (NWB), or partially in partial-weight-bearing (PWB) mode.

For non-weight-bearing walking, you place the crutches a short way in front of you, splaying them slightly outwards to give yourself room, then take your weight through your hands and hop forwards on your uninjured leg so that you land level with or slightly in front of the crutches. In partial weight-bearing put the crutches forward, press on your hands and take the injured leg forward level with the crutches, then step through to place the uninjured leg level with or slightly in front of the crutches. Never put the crutches too far away from you, especially in wet conditions, as they might skid. Pay attention as you walk: avoid being distracted, looking round or rushing.

Stairs

Going up stairs, legs go first, crutches afterwards: hop or step up to put your uninjured leg on the stair above, then bring the crutches up to the same level. To go down stairs, the crutches go first: place the crutches down on the step in front of you, then hop on your uninjured leg or step down with your injured leg to the same level. Always make sure you place the crutches in the centre of each step, not close to the edge. For more stability and better balance on stairs, use one crutch and the bannister or rail.

Progressive weight-bearing

From non-weight-bearing, you gradually progress to partial-weight-bearing as your injury recovers. If you have used crutches for some time, you have to wean off them gradually. You need to be able to take close to your full weight through the injured leg before you progress to using one crutch or a walking stick, which should be held on the opposite side to the injured leg. Keep using a support until your leg can take all of your body weight and you can walk absolutely normally without problems.

Exercises for walking, to correct or prevent a limp

These exercises should be done following any leg injury which has made you limp. Use a support or crutches as necessary. Do the exercises in front of a mirror at first, to make sure you are doing them correctly.

Early stage exercises

1. Sitting or standing with your feet parallel and slightly apart, lift one heel up, lower it, then lift the other. Keep the pressure over the ball of the foot, and do not let the foot splay inwards or outwards. 10–20 times. Gradually increase the speed.

2. Standing up straight with your good leg on a support level with the top of the weighing scale, place the foot of your injured leg flat on a weighing scale; press down on the scale as much as you can without discomfort, keeping your knee and body as straight as possible, head up and shoulders level. Repeat 3–5 times, and record your highest score. Practise regularly until you can take your whole body weight through the injured leg.

3. Standing with your good leg on the floor, place the ball of the foot of your injured leg on a weighing scale, with your knee bent; keeping the knee bent and heel up, press down on the scale as much as you can without discomfort, with your head up, shoulders level and good leg straight. Repeat 3–5 times, and record your highest score. Practise regularly until you can take your whole body weight through the injured leg.

4. Standing in front of a mirror with feet parallel and slightly apart, shift your weight slightly sideways over your injured leg, and raise the shoulder on that side upwards a little way, keeping your arms by your sides, knees straight and your feet on the floor. 5 times.

5. With your good leg on a support level with the top of the weighing scale, place the ball of the foot of your injured leg on the weighing scale, with your knee straight; press down on the scale as much as you can without discomfort, keeping your knee and body straight, head up and shoulders level. Repeat 3–5 times, and record your highest score. Practise regularly until you can take your whole body weight through the injured leg.

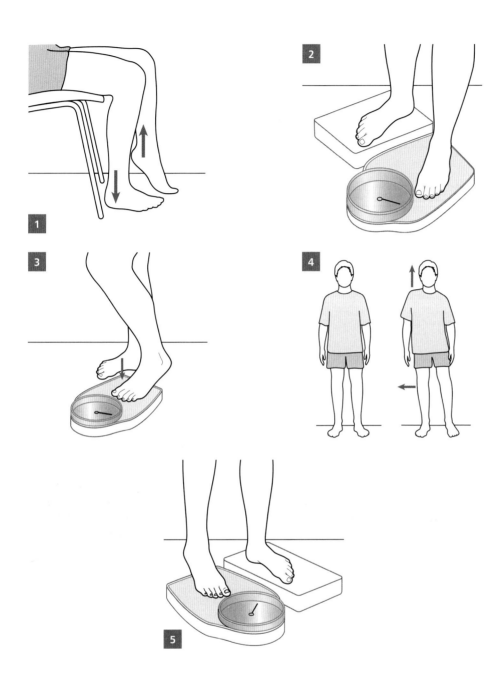

Balance exercises

Stand beside a support at first. When you can do the first exercise easily, you can start doing the others as well. As your balance improves, you can use a wobble board, rocker board, mini-trampoline or BOSU (diagram 6) to make the exercises more demanding.

1. Standing on your injured leg, hold your balance for as long as you can, then relax for a count of 10. 3–5 times.

2. Standing on your injured leg, lift your arms up and down in all directions for as long as you can keep your balance, then relax for a count of 10. 3 times.

3. Standing on your injured leg, lift the other leg out sideways and round in circles until you lose your balance, then relax for a count of 10. 3 times.

4. Standing on your injured leg, throw a ball up in the air and catch it as many times as you can while holding your balance, then relax for a count of 10. 3 times. Variation: throw the ball against a wall or to a partner.

5. Standing on your injured leg, close your eyes and hold your balance, then relax for a count of 10. 3–5 times.

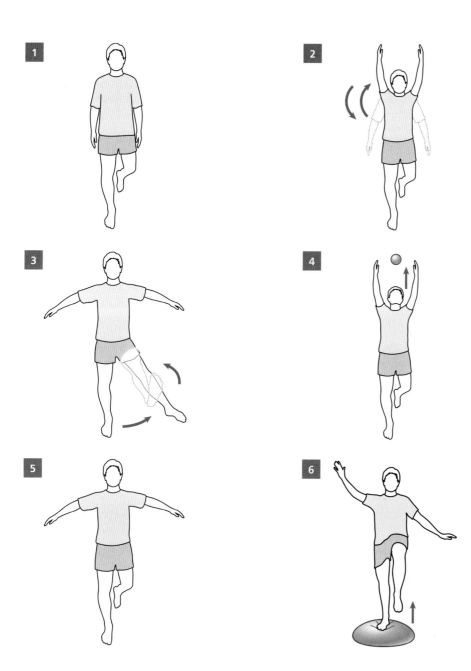

Advanced walking exercises

1. Standing with your feet parallel and slightly apart, go up on your toes, keeping your weight over the balls of the feet and your knees locked straight; using your hips, shift your weight slightly over the injured side, return to centre and then lower your heels. 10 times.

2. Standing, shift your weight slightly sideways over your injured leg and lift the arm on that side upwards to reach above your head; lift the opposite leg out to the side, move it inwards and outwards 3 times without putting the foot down, then return to the starting position. 5 times.

3. High stepping: put one foot forward and lift the heel immediately to go up on your toes as you bring the other leg through the air. 10–20 steps.

4. Walk backwards: stand up straight and take steps backwards. Start slowly and gradually build up speed. 20–30 steps. Variation: walk backwards in a figure-of-eight pattern.

5. Walk sideways: take a step to the side and bring the other foot up to the leading foot. 20–30 steps in each direction. Start slowly and gradually build up speed.

6. Walk sideways with cross-over: take a step to the side with one foot; bring the other foot across in front of the leading foot. Start slowly and gradually build up speed. 20–30 steps in each direction. Variation: take the trail foot behind the leading foot.

7. Standing, roll your feet outwards into supination, lifting the inner arch; take steps forwards, backwards and sideways, keeping your weight on the outer edges of your feet. 20–30 steps.

8. Standing, lift your toes and forefoot to take steps in all directions, walking on your heels. 20–30 steps.

9. Standing on one leg, go up and down on your toes, keeping the weight over the ball of the foot, knee locked straight, head up and shoulders level. 3–5 times.

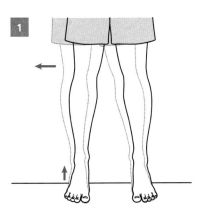
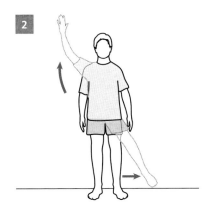

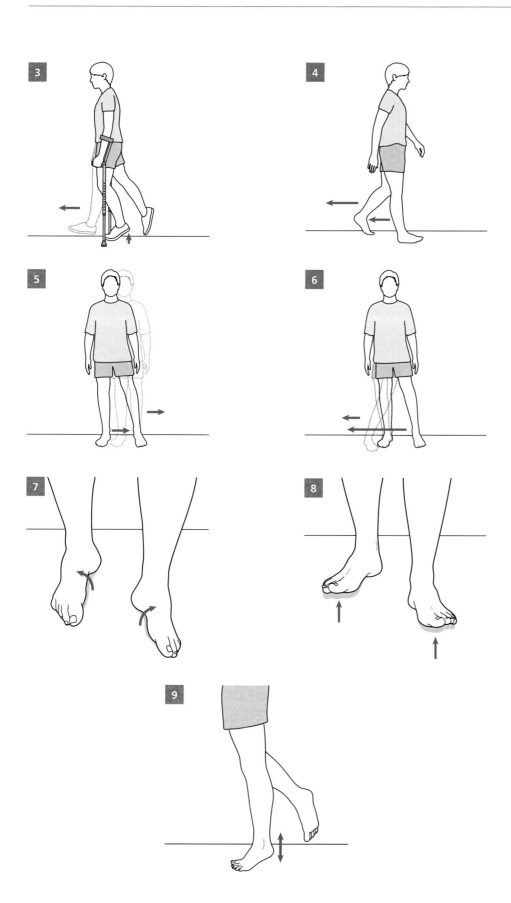

4

The Foot

RIGHT FOOT, SEEN OBLIQUELY FROM THE INNER (MEDIAL) SIDE.

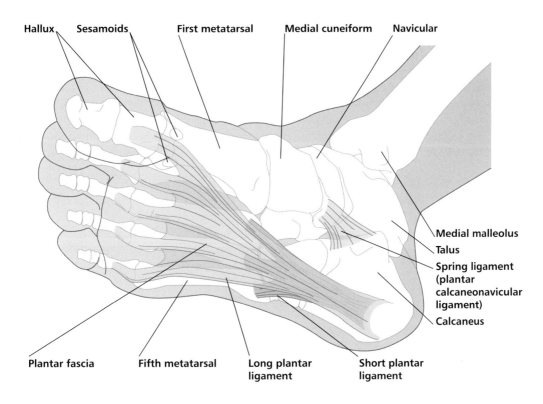

The foot is the end point of the leg and consists of 26 small bones.

Structure

Bones and joints

Seven bones at the back of the foot and under the ankle, including the calcaneus (heel bone) form the tarsus. The talus lies on top of the front of the calcaneus; the cuboid is on the outer side of the talus, the navicular in front of it; beside the cuboid is the lateral cuneiform, next to which are the intermediate and medial cuneiforms, which lie in front of the navicular.

The five bones leading towards the toes form the metatarsus. They are numbered from the inner side of the foot, so the metatarsal leading to the big toe is the first, and the one to the little toe the fifth.

The big toe (hallux) consists of two bones called phalanges, which are thicker and stronger than the three which form each of the four smaller toes. There are two tiny floating bones called sesamoids under the ball of the big toe, which are held in place by tendons.

The foot bones are linked together as synovial joints, with capsules, ligaments and synovial membranes. Within the intertarsal joints, the main part of the joint between the talus and calcaneus is known as the subtalar joint, while the front forms the talocalcaneonavicular joint. The metatarsal bones are connected to the hindfoot in plane joints, while their connections to the toes are classified as ellipsoid. The interphalangeal toe joints are hinge joints.

Of the many ligaments which bind the foot bones together, two are especially important. The 'spring' ligament links the calcaneus to the navicular, and helps to support the medial arch. The long plantar ligament extends from the calcaneus across the cuboid to the near ends or bases of the middle three metatarsals. It helps support the lateral arch. The plantar fascia is a strong band which binds the structures under the sole of your foot, and separates the skin from the muscles and tendons.

Muscles and tendons

The foot contains small muscles called the intrinsics, which lie between the bones, forming four layers under the sole and a single layer over the top (dorsum) of the foot.

On the top of the foot is the extensor digitorum brevis, which runs from the navicular to the top of the first part of the big toe and the second to fourth toes. The deepest-lying muscles under the foot (the fourth layer) are the dorsal and plantar interossei, which connect the metatarsals to the nearer ends of the toes. The next, third layer consists of flexor hallucis brevis between the cuboid, lateral cuneiform and the first part of the big toe, whose two tendons contain the sesamoid bones; adductor hallucis, connecting the second to fourth metatarsals with the outer sesamoid (close to the second toe) and the base of the first part of the big toe; and flexor digiti minimi brevis, which runs from the base of the fifth metatarsal to the first part of the fifth toe. The second layer consists of flexor digitorum accessorius, which connects the calcaneus to the long flexor tendons, and the lumbrical muscles, which also connect to the flexor digitorum longus tendons and are fixed to the near ends of the second to fifth toes. The first layer, closest to the surface of the sole, consists of abductor hallucis, which runs from the calcaneus to the inner side of the base of the near end of the big toe; flexor digitorum brevis, between the calcaneus and the underside of the ends of the toes; and abductor digiti minimi, which runs between the calcaneus and the base of the near end of the little toe.

Longer muscles from the lower leg also act on the foot and toes (pp. 85–86), including tibialis anterior, the long toe extensors and peroneus tertius over the front; peronei longus and brevis on the outer side; and tibialis posterior, the long toe flexors and the Achilles tendon (p. 70) from behind. Where the tendons pass close to the ankle they are protected in fluid-producing synovial sheaths which help provide friction-free movements.

Variations

Within the basic structure of the bones and soft tissues there are individual differences. Some you are born with, others develop through use, injury or aging. Your heel might be relatively narrow and your forefoot wide, and vice versa. If the second toe is longer than the big toe (hallux), it is called a 'Morton's foot'. Toes can be extra long or short, stiff, pliable or dextrous. The inner arch can be unusually raised in a high-arched foot, which is often associated with bow leg at the knee, or dropped towards the ground in a so-called 'flat foot', which can be linked to knock-knee or in-turned hip.

Functions

The foot bones form functional arches which transmit forces during weight-bearing movements like walking and running. The inner side or instep of the sole forms the medial longitudinal arch and is normally higher than the outer (lateral) arch, which is flatter and closer to the ground.

The foot is pliable, and adapts to uneven surfaces through proprioception. It becomes more rigid when you sprint or jump. You pivot over it in dancing or sports like squash and field hockey. It absorbs the shock when your foot lands on the ground during running or jumping. It strengthens for sports like football and contact martial arts. With training, the foot can also perform delicate tasks normally performed by the hand, such as drawing.

Patterns of weight-bearing

When you walk or run, weight is transmitted from the outer edge of the heel, along the lateral arch, then over to the ball of the foot behind the big toe. Hardened skin forms for protection, so most often there is a calloused area under the ball of the foot. In a 'Morton's foot' the callous pad forms under the head of the second toe. Some people walk and run on the outer edges of the feet: this is called 'oversupination', and is usually caused by tightness in the tibialis anterior, sometimes together with altered mechanics of the knees and hips. Rolling your feet inwards as you walk or run, flattening the medial arch, is called 'overpronation'. This is usually caused by tibialis anterior weakness, often coupled with poor mechanics in the leg up to the hip.

Muscle actions

When you are standing, tibialis anterior helps to keep the leg in position over the ankle. Together with peroneus longus, it stabilizes the medial arch of the foot, especially when you tiptoe, or in the push-off phase of running.

Supination is part of the movement called 'inversion', in which you turn the inner edge of the foot upwards, lifting the medial arch. The movement is performed by tibialis anterior and posterior, which normally prevent overpronation when you walk or run. Pronation is part of the opposite movement of 'eversion', which is performed by the peronei, longus and brevis. These movements take place mainly in the subtalar joint.

The four outer toes curl downwards into flexion against a resistance or gravity through the action of the lumbricals, interossei, flexor digitorum muscles (longus and brevis) and flexor digiti minimi brevis. The big toe is flexed by its long and short flexors.

The outer toes are drawn upwards into extension by the extensor digitorum muscles, the big toe by extensor hallucis longus. The big toe is drawn towards the other foot into abduction through the action of abductor hallucis, and into adduction towards the second toe by adductor hallucis, while the third to fifth toes are moved inwards towards the second toe by the first, second and third plantar interossei. The dorsal interossei abduct the toes.

Shoes

The human foot is designed to function barefoot. We wear shoes to protect the foot against rain and cold, and to prevent skin damage. Shoes must never block the feet. They should be flexible, not rigid.

Fit

Your shoes should be big enough to allow your feet to spread as you walk or run, without causing pressure or friction. The upper should have as few seams as possible.

The toe-box should be broader than the heel area. The heel counter should fit snugly round the calcaneus. It should be vertical at the back (sideways on), and should end at ankle level. A heel tab above ankle level can damage the lower end of the Achilles tendon (p. 75). With the laces done up, the shoe or boot should feel comfortably stable.

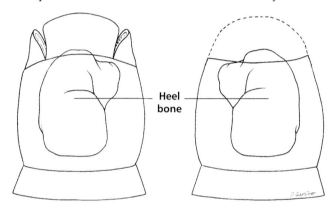

Heel bone

The shoe back should be no higher than the heel bone.

Sole

The sole should conform to the upper of the shoe. A narrow sole makes the foot unstable: excess width throws the foot off-balance. The sole should be flexible from the midfoot forward. The only firm part should be directly under the heel.

You need different soles for natural and artificial surfaces, or if the conditions are wet or dry. For sports which are played on varied surfaces, you need several pairs of shoes.

Insole

The insole is important for cushioning. Check your insoles regularly for undue wear, and change them immediately: this can extend the life of your sports shoes. If your foot mechanics need correcting, an orthotic insole fitted by a podiatrist is best.

Choosing shoes

1. Look at the shoe from all angles making sure it is foot-shaped.

2. Feel inside for seams or protruding parts.

3. Bend the shoe in all directions to check that it is flexible.

4. Put the shoes on, with your sports socks and insoles; stand up, go up and down on your toes, then jog around in them.

5. Make sure your feet have plenty of space.

6. Shoe sizes vary, so be guided by the feel of the shoe, and take a bigger size than usual if necessary.

Pain and complications

Causes of gradual or unexplained pain in one or both feet include inflammatory joint problems such as rheumatoid arthritis, gout, diabetes, ankylosing spondylitis (p. 170), thyroid problems, circulatory problems, reflex sympathetic dystrophy (p. 10), neurological conditions, and referred symptoms from the leg, hip or back. 'Dropped foot' (p. 94) or inability to control your foot movements properly can arise from 'trapped nerve' problems in your back (p. 219), or can be a complication of hip replacement surgery.

Foot injuries

The bones and soft tissues of the foot can be injured through trauma or overuse at any age. Any foot injury has a direct effect on the whole leg, and can cause overload on the opposite side through limping.

Skin conditions

Hard skin under the foot is protective, so it is best not to remove it. Hard skin and blisters over the top of the feet usually mean that your shoes are too tight, or your socks are chafing.

Skin care
Look after the skin of your feet: keep your feet clean; use soft absorbent socks and wash them after each use; always leave your sports shoes out to air after use; and cover any open wounds with sticking plaster or clean dressings. Wear protective footwear in shared changing and shower rooms, to avoid getting or spreading contagions like verrucas or athlete's foot. If you get a skin infection, have it dealt with promptly by your doctor, chiropodist or podiatrist.

Traumatic fracture

Any of the bones in the foot can be broken or cracked in a sudden traumatic injury. This can happen at any age. In adolescents trauma can damage the epiphyseal plate or growth area within a bone. This is particularly common in the metatarsals, and is called Freiberg's condition. It can lead to bone weakness and the formation of bone fragments (loose bodies).

What you feel
Pain can be severe or slight at the moment of injury. There may be bleeding if the bone is badly disrupted. Even if the bone is not displaced, there is usually swelling and bruising round the injury, and you may notice numbness or tingling sensations. Weight-bearing hurts, although you may be able to walk with a limp. When your foot is off the ground, the foot may or may not hurt. Aching builds up if you sit or stand still for a length of time.

Causes
Jarring or a sudden shock from a fall or direct blow can break the foot bones. Contributory factors include tight, stiff shoes and wearing shoes with the wrong grip for the playing surface, especially on artificial surfaces. If the bones are weak through dietary insufficiency or osteoporosis, fractures happen more easily.

Directions
Your foot may be immobilized in a splint or plaster cast, and you should use crutches. If the fracture is complicated, you may be offered an operation to stabilize the bones.

How long?
3–12 months.

Stress fracture

Any bone in the foot can crack through overuse stress (p. 6). It can happen at any age, but is most common in teenagers and young adults. One possible complication of a navicular stress fracture in children under the age of ten is avascular necrosis, or loss of the blood supply to the bone, which is known as Köhler's disease.

What you feel
The first sign is usually an ache over the bone after exercising, or later on in bed at night. If you rest for a few days, the pain goes away, but returns if you resume the same training. If you continue, the pain gradually gets worse, so much so that even walking hurts. The bone is tender if you press it. You may notice slight swelling.

Causes
Repetitive stress, mainly due to muscles or tendons pulling on the bone, causes micro-trauma. Biomechanics are a bigger factor than simple jarring. You may have increased your running mileage, resumed training after a lay-off, or done intensive sessions of rope skipping or hopping and bounding. If you are normally sedentary you can be at risk if you go on long hikes over several days without proper preparation.

Which bone is affected depends on your style of walking or running and your activities. For instance in 'Morton's foot' a stress fracture can happen in the second metatarsal head which leads into the second toe, whereas if you tend to oversupinate, turning the foot outwards, the fourth or fifth metatarsal heads are more vulnerable.

Stress fractures happen in healthy bone. They happen more easily when bones are weakened by dietary deficiency, osteoporosis or disease.

Directions
You should not need a cast, although sometimes immobilization in a walking cast is used for a child, especially if there is a complication such as Köhler's disease. Avoid repetitive or painful activities for as long as it takes for the bone to heal. Do pain-free alternative training to stimulate healing. You may be able to cycle. Metatarsals usually heal within six weeks, while the thicker bones, such as the calcaneus and the midfoot, can take up to three months. Allow two weeks after healing before gradually resuming your sport.

How long?
2–6 months.

Soft tissue strain

Any of the foot's ligaments, muscles or tendons can be torn, partly torn or strained through trauma or overuse at any age.

What you feel
Even minimal soft tissue damage can be extremely painful. Pain is usually felt on a specific movement, especially when your weight is on the foot. It may be worse barefoot or in certain shoes, or when you walk or run on a particular surface or uneven ground.

There may be localized or general swelling. There is usually tenderness, for instance under the medial arch if the 'spring' ligament is damaged. With muscle or tendon injury, you feel pain when it contracts or is stretched.

There is usually little or no pain at rest, but your foot may stiffen up if you sit or lie still for long periods.

Causes
Gradual pain is often related to ill-fitting or stiff shoes. If your shoes fit snugly, they may become tight during sport, for instance in long-distance running or a lengthy tennis match in hot conditions. Your feet tend to swell more on synthetic playing surfaces. A sudden strain can be caused by an awkward movement or catching the foot, perhaps on the edge of a step, a stone, or rough ground.

Directions
Correct or discard any shoes which are uncomfortable. You may be offered orthotics to support the foot in the correct position.

How long?
1–6 months.

Metatarsalgia

This is a general term describing pain in the forefoot between the metatarsal heads which lead into the toes. It can come on gradually or suddenly, and can happen at any age, although it is probably least common among children.

What you feel
There is pain in the forefoot when your weight is on it, especially when you run or jump. There is usually little or no pain at rest.

Causes
Shoes which are too tight across the toes are the most common cause, especially if they also have rigid soles. Another possible factor is alteration in your foot movements, perhaps due to painful blisters, a leg injury, new shoes or a change in your running or jumping technique.

Directions
Identify and correct the cause.

How long?
5 days to several months.

Interdigital neuroma

Interdigital neuroma, or Morton's metatarsalgia, is a condition in which a nerve is compressed between two metatarsal heads and swells up in a painful lump. It can happen at any age, but is rare in children.

What you feel
There is a very localized sharp pain in the forefoot when the foot is in a certain position, usually with your weight on it. The pain can be relieved instantly if you remove your shoe and rub your foot.

Causes
A shoe which is too narrow and tight is the most common cause, but a change in foot mechanics is another possible factor.

Directions
Identify the cause, and correct or discard any faulty shoes. If the pain is severe, you may be offered an injection or an operation.

How long?
10 days to several weeks.

Tenosynovitis

Swelling in the fluid-lined synovial sheaths which protect tendons is called tenosynovitis. The top (dorsum) of the foot from the front of the ankle is especially vulnerable to this problem, which can happen at any age, but is least common among young children.

What you feel
A swollen area marks out the shape of the tendon sheath over the top of the foot, and you feel a grating sensation when you move the foot or toes up and down. The foot feels stiff when you point it downwards. There is pain if your shoes rub the swollen area.

Causes
The problem can occur suddenly from a direct blow to the top of the foot. More often it is an overuse problem due to excessive repetitive movements, usually combined with friction from your shoe. Sometimes the tongue of the shoe is poorly shaped or too thin.

Directions
Make sure your shoes do not chafe. Modify or discard any which cause irritation.

How long?
2–6 weeks.

Plantar fasciitis

The plantar fascia under the sole of the foot can be partly torn or strained. This can happen suddenly, but is usually a gradual problem which affects one or both feet. It can happen at any age, but is especially common in middle-aged men.

What you feel
There is a dull or sharp pain under the foot, which either spreads the length of the foot or concentrates in the spot where the plantar fascia joins the calcaneus. If you press it, the painful area feels tender. You feel pain when you go up on your toes and stretch the sole of the foot. In some cases, just putting your foot to the floor causes pain, especially if you have been sitting or lying down for some time. Usually there is no pain when you are at rest with no pressure on your foot.

Causes
Stiff-soled shoes are a common cause, alongside altered foot biomechanics. The pain can be caused or influenced by various inflammatory conditions: for instance, in teenage boys it can be a symptom of ankylosing spondylitis (p. 170). Hormonal changes can play a part.

Directions
Discard any shoes which cause discomfort. Arch supports may help, and you may benefit from custom-fitted supportive orthotics. If the pain is severe, your doctor may offer an injection.

How long?
1 week to several months.

Heel bruise

The fat pad under the heel becomes painful and inflamed. This can be a sudden or, less often, a gradual injury, and can happen at any age.

What you feel
There is pain under the heel on direct pressure when the heel strikes the ground or if you prod it hard. There is usually little or no pain at rest.

Causes
Most often a heel bruise is caused by a sudden jarring, perhaps from stamping, or on landing hard from a jump. It can be caused by repetitive pressure on the heel, for instance in long-distance running. Shoes with hard or worn soles and hard playing or running surfaces can contribute.

Directions
Protect the heel with soft padding, and avoid taking weight through it until the acute phase passes. You may be offered orthotics.

How long?
Up to several weeks.

Heel bursitis

The small sac of fluid which lies between the Achilles tendon and the back of the heel becomes inflamed. Bursitis can also occur under the heel. It is usually an overuse injury, and can happen at any age.

What you feel
There is pain on direct pressure, but little or no pain when you stand barefoot and go up and down on your toes.

Causes
Most often heel bursitis is caused by friction from hard, worn, badly shaped or ill-fitting shoes. Sometimes it is associated with repetitive forceful foot and ankle movements, for instance through practising floor exercises in gymnastics.

Directions
Discard any faulty shoes. You may need to put padding inside the back of your shoe or round the edges of the sole to reduce direct pressure on the heel. For severe pain, you may be offered an injection.

How long?
Up to several weeks.

Heel spur

A small spike of bone forms, growing out from the calcaneus, most often under the sole of the foot where the plantar fascia joins the heel. The spur forms over a long space of time, so it is mainly seen in adults.

What you feel
The spur may or may not cause pain. A painless spur may be found incidentally on an X-ray for another injury. A painful spur usually hurts when the sole of the foot is stretched, and it may be tender if you prod it hard.

Causes
The spur results from attrition at the attachment point where the soft tissue meets the bone. Shoes with hard, stiff soles or insufficient arch support, unforgiving playing or running surfaces, and faulty foot biomechanics can all play a part.

Directions
Check your shoes, and put padding round the heel area to reduce pressure. You may benefit from arch supports or custom-fitted orthotics. In a chronic case you may be offered surgery.

How long?
2 weeks to several months.

Calcaneal apophysitis

The back edge of the calcaneus does not unite properly with the main part of the bone. This is an overuse problem which happens during growth in childhood, usually between the ages of ten and sixteen. It is often referred to as Sever's 'disease' or calcaneal epiphysitis. The injury is very similar to a stress fracture (p. 46).

What you feel
There is gradually increasing pain at the back of the heel in sports like soccer, netball, tennis gymnastics and running. The bone is tender to touch and may feel inflamed. There is usually no pain at rest at first, although there may be pain at night.

Causes
The usual cause is repetitive jarring, combined with the pull of the Achilles tendon, especially during a growth spurt. Stiff shoes and hard playing surfaces can contribute.

Directions
Rest from repetitive or painful activities which stress the foot for as long as it takes for the bone to heal fully. Meanwhile you should do painless exercises and alternative training to stimulate the circulation. You may benefit from cushioning heel pads, but should not need a cast.

How long?
6–12 weeks.

Sesamoid injury

The sesamoid bones under the ball of the foot can be injured through trauma, causing one or both bones to split, crack or suffer bruising. Overuse injury can cause a stress fracture (p. 46) in one or occasionally both bones. If there is inflammation in the area without particular bone damage, it is called sesamoiditis. Occasionally diagnosis is complicated by the fact that some people have double sesamoids which look as though they have split when they have not. Sesamoid problems can happen at any age.

What you feel
Putting pressure over the ball of the foot is painful, especially if you twist or pivot, as in standing on tiptoe and turning to one side, sprinting, skipping or hopping. There may be pain shortly after weight-bearing activities, but at rest there is usually little or no pain.

Causes
Traumatic injury can result from jumping on to a hard surface and landing awkwardly on the ball of the foot, especially if your shoes have hard or thin soles. Running and turning can cause the injury if your shoes have too much grip for the playing surface.

Overuse injury can be caused by persistent jarring and adverse stress, often through doing a lot of sport in inappropriate shoes or on an unfamiliar surface.

Directions

Discard any shoes which cause discomfort. You may benefit from arch supports or custom-fitted orthotics. Your doctor may offer an injection. In a chronic case you may be offered surgery.

How long?

2 weeks to several months.

Bunion

A bunion is a deformity at the base of the big toe. It usually develops slowly and gradually. The big toe is pulled towards the second toe, so that its joint with the first metatarsal bone is forced outwards, forming a lumpy protrusion on the side of the foot. Technically this is called hallux valgus. There may be localized swelling or bursitis over the lump. The problem is much more common in females than males. It is rare in young children, but the first signs may appear in the teens.

What you feel

A bunion may or may not be painful when you put weight on your foot. It is rarely painful when there is no pressure on it. Very often the main complaint is that the bunion looks unsightly and makes it difficult to find shoes which fit comfortably.

Causes

The muscles and tendons controlling the big toe become unbalanced, with weakness in those which hold the big toe away from the other toes. Very often bunions are caused by narrow-fronted shoes. Women's high heels with pointed toes are a particular problem. Classical ballerinas often suffer from bunions because of pointe shoes, or the abnormal pattern of walking which results from having the hips permanently turned out. Bunions can be hereditary, or linked to diseases like rheumatoid arthritis.

Directions

Discard any shoes which are tight over the forefoot. Arch supports or custom-fitted orthotics may help. In a severe case, you may need surgery.

How long?

After surgery: 3–9 months.
Without surgery: the bunion may remain fairly prominent, but any pain should reduce within weeks with exercises and treatment.

Hammer toes

This is a gradual process in which the toes become deformed, lifting up at their central joints and pressing down at the tips. It may be associated with a high arch in the foot. It is most common in adults from middle to older age, but can happen earlier. In young children it can be associated with spasticity, usually from a congenital condition.

What you feel
The condition usually causes little or no pain in itself, unless chafing from shoes causes blisters and soreness.

Causes
The tendons leading into the toes become tight, either because of ill-fitting shoes, or through overwork or compensation mechanisms, for instance if the calf muscles or other parts of the leg have been weakened by injury, making you walk awkwardly.

Directions
Make sure all your shoes allow adequate room in the forefoot. You may benefit from custom-fitted orthotics. If the problem is too advanced for exercises alone to help, you may need surgery.

How long?
After surgery: 3–6 months.
Without surgery: this is a long-term problem, but you may be able to continue your normal sports despite the deformity.

Hallux rigidus

The big toe joint progressively stiffens in a gradual process which affects mainly adults.

What you feel
Movement in the big toe becomes limited, sometimes painful if you force it. There may be pain when the big toe is under pressure in activities like sprinting, hopping, and landing from a jump, or if you wear tight or stiff-soled shoes.

Causes
Most often the stiffness follows a jarring injury to the big toe, especially if the injury happened during childhood or adolescent growth phases. The stiffness may come on long after the injury. Sometimes the problem is caused by wearing stiff-soled shoes.

Directions
Discard any stiff shoes, and make sure all your shoes have enough room to allow your toes to spread. You may benefit from arch supports or custom-fitted orthotics. In a severe case, you may be offered an operation.

How long?
1–6 months.

The Foot

Black toenails

Damage to the toes can cause bleeding or bruising under the nail, which makes the toe look black. The problem can be traumatic or gradual, and can happen at any age.

What you feel
There is usually little pain, but you may have a feeling of pressure under the nail.

Causes
Traumatic injury can be caused by a direct blow to the toe nail, for instance if a weight drops on to the foot, or through kicking a football awkwardly. Gradual injury can happen as a result of shoes or boots which are tight over the toes, or have seams which catch the nails.

Directions
Discard any shoes which cause pressure or friction over the toes. Always cut your nails evenly, straight across the tops of the toes. You can release the blood from under the nail by piercing vertically down through the nail with a sterilized needle, but it is better to seek help from your doctor, chiropodist or podiatrist.

Once the bruising under the nail has been released, the nail will grow through normally, although this may take several months. In some cases, the nail may remain thicker and harder than the other nails. In older age it may need chiropody treatment to keep it trim.

How long?
This problem should not interfere with your sport.

Rehabilitation and recovery

Acute phase

Use the circulatory care measures (p. 27) and crutches according to your practitioner's instructions. Alternative training for the unaffected parts of your body should start as soon as possible (p. 25).

Early phase

As soon as you can, when your practitioner allows, you should do foot exercises such as those listed below to regain precise movements, coordination, muscle action and mobility in the injured foot. Always work within pain limits. The exercises are best done barefoot, but you can use soft flexible shoes if you prefer. The exercises should be combined with non-weight-bearing ankle exercises (p. 66) and early stage walking exercises (p. 34). For the standing-up exercises, you may need to use crutches or a support at first. Do the exercises on the non-injured foot as well, but do more repetitions on the injured side. Aim for at least one session a day, preferably two or three. You must recover good strength and efficiency in the small muscles of the foot before progressing to more demanding exercises.

Recovery phase

When you can take weight through the foot, you need to do balance exercises (p. 36) and advanced walking exercises (p. 38). The correct pattern for weight-bearing is a priority. You should also do strengthening exercises for the calf (p. 82), front thigh (p. 127), hamstrings (p. 136), inner thigh (p. 146) and hip (p. 162). You must recover good balance and soleus function (p. 82, exercise 4) before progressing to the final recovery phase (p. 308).

Foot strengthening exercises

1. Sitting or standing with your feet flat on the floor, press your toes gently down, keeping them straight and flat against the floor; hold for a count of 5, then relax completely. 3–6 times.

2. Sitting or standing with your feet flat on the floor, press your big toe down into the floor, keeping it straight and flat, and holding the other toes slightly off the floor; hold for a count of 5, then relax. 3–6 times.

3. Sitting or standing with your toes on the edge of a weighing scale and the rest of the foot supported at the same height, press your toes flat on to the scale without letting your toes curl. Repeat 5 times, and record your highest score.

4. Sitting or standing with your feet flat on the floor, spread all your toes sideways to separate them, keeping them flat and in contact with the floor. 5–10 times.

5. Sitting or standing, spread your big toe to the side, away from the second toe, keeping it flat on the floor. 5–10 times.

6. Sitting or standing, roll your foot outwards to lift the inner (medial) arch up slightly, keeping your toes and heel in contact with the floor, and your legs still (press against your knees to prevent your legs from moving if necessary). 5–10 times, first on each foot separately, then both feet together symmetrically.

7. Sitting on a chair, barefoot, place a pencil on the floor and curl your toes to grip it; a) lift your toes and the pencil upwards, keeping your heel down; b) grip the pencil and lift the whole leg, bend and straighten your knee in the air, then put the foot and pencil down again. Repeat each sequence 3–5 times.

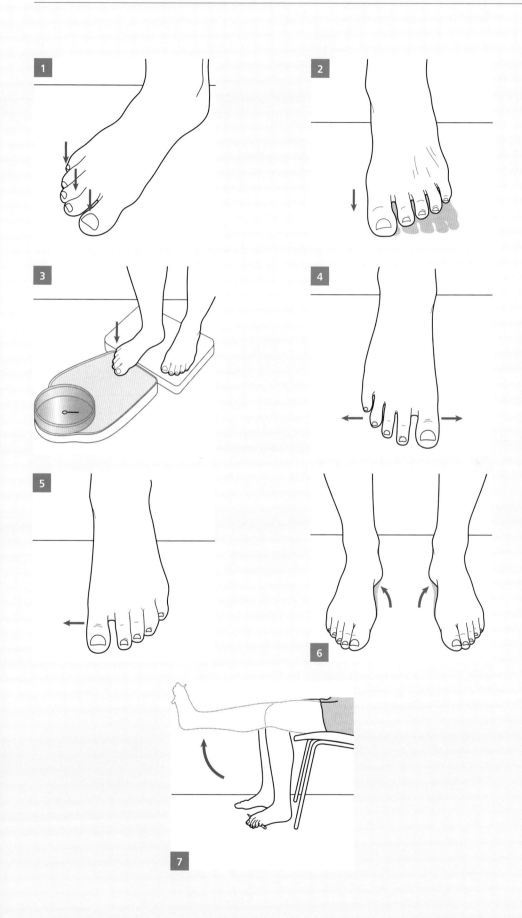

The Foot

Foot mobilizing and stretching exercises

1. Sitting on a chair, rest the arch of your foot on a small ball – such as a golf ball – and move your foot around to massage it over the ball. Do this as often and for as long as you like.

2. Lying on your stomach, tuck your toes under to lift your heels up, then straighten your knees as hard as you can to stretch the soles of your feet; hold for a count of 6, then relax completely. 5 times with both legs working together, then 5 times on each leg separately.

3. Sitting or standing, stretch the sole of your foot by pressing your toes against a vertical surface and bending your ankle to take your knee forward over the foot, keeping your heel in contact with the floor; hold for a count of 6, then relax completely. 5–10 times.

4. Sitting, stretch the top of your foot by pressing the toes and foot downwards with your hand or the other foot; hold for a count of 6, then relax completely. 5–10 times.

5. Kneeling, with legs slightly apart and parallel, and the tops of your feet in contact with the floor, sit back on your heels keeping your feet in contact with the floor; hold for a count of 6, then relax completely. 5–10 times.

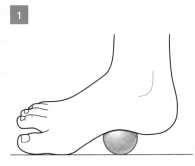

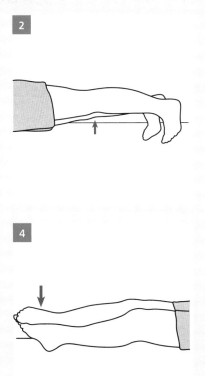

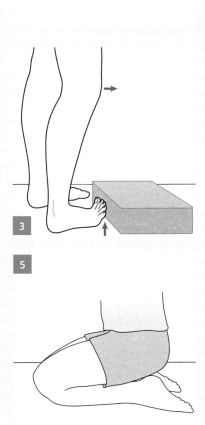

5

The Ankle

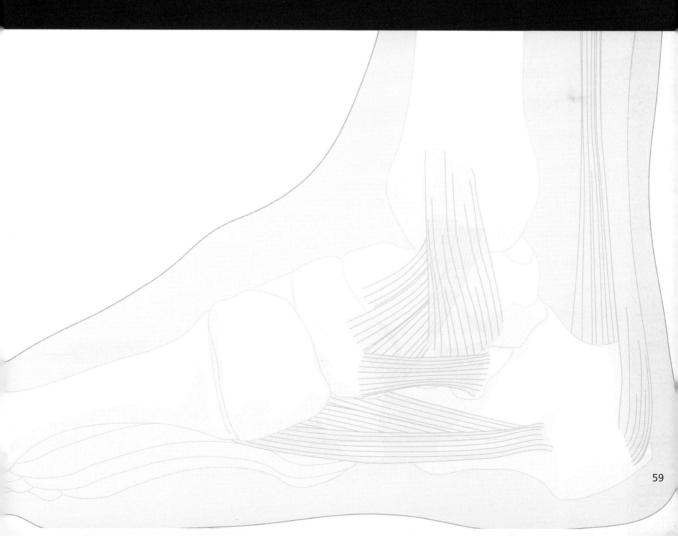

RIGHT FOOT AND ANKLE, SEEN FROM THE INNER (MEDIAL) SIDE.

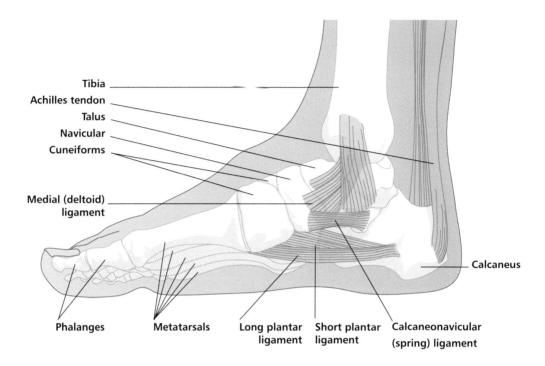

Tibia

Achilles tendon

Talus

Navicular

Cuneiforms

Medial (deltoid) ligament

Calcaneus

Phalanges   Metatarsals   Long plantar ligament   Short plantar ligament   Calcaneonavicular (spring) ligament

The ankle, or talocrural joint, connects the foot to the leg, and is basically a hinge joint.

Structure

Bones

Three bones form the ankle: the talus, tibia (shinbone) and fibula (outer leg bone). The lower ends of the tibia and fibula form an inverted U shape over the talus. On either side of the ankle you can see and feel the bony points (malleoli) at the ends of the bones. The subtalar joint lies under the ankle, formed by the underside of the talus and the top of the front part of the calcaneus (heel bone).

Soft tissues

The ankle joint is bound within its fibrous capsule, which is lined by a fluid-producing synovial membrane. The capsule is strengthened by strong ligaments on either side of the ankle – the medial deltoid ligament on the inner side, and the lateral ligament on the outer side, part of which also protects the back of the joint. The front of the joint is the least protected. The tibia and fibula are bound together above the ankle by the inferior (lower) tibiofibular, or transverse, ligament.

Muscles from the lower leg pass downwards across the ankle (p. 86). Over the front are tibialis anterior, the toe extensors and peroneus tertius, while at the back are tibialis posterior, the long toe flexors and the Achilles tendon (p. 71), with the peronei longus and brevis (p. 85) to the outer side. Where tendons lie close to the ankle, they are held in place by strong bands called retinacula, and protected from friction by tube-like sheaths filled with synovial fluid.

The ankle has a rich supply of proprioceptive nerves, which are vital for your balance mechanisms when you are standing or moving about on your feet.

Functions

The ankle allows the foot to move up and down. Although the ankle has a slight degree of sideways and twisting movements when the foot is pointing downwards, these are accessory movements, which you cannot perform at will. The foot's twisting and rotation movements occur in the subtalar and foot joints, not the ankle.

The tendons around the ankle create movements, as well as acting to stabilize and protect the joint. Against gravity, a resistance or your body weight, gastrocnemius and soleus point your foot downwards into plantarflexion, helped by plantaris, the long toe flexors and tibialis posterior if necessary. Tibialis anterior brings the top of the foot up at the ankle into dorsiflexion, and turns the foot inwards and slightly upwards into inversion. The long toe extensors and peroneus tertius help the movement when more pressure is needed.

When you stand still, the line of gravity falls just in front of your ankle joint, so the postural muscles, especially soleus, are constantly adjusting slightly to keep you upright. When you walk, run or jump, the ankle is the link for movement and shock absorption between your foot and lower leg. The load of your body weight is transmitted through the tibia on to the surface of the talus. The fibula does not take your body weight, but moves very slightly outwards as your leg goes forwards over the talus.

Pain and complications

Unexplained or unusual pain or swelling in the ankle can be caused by infection (p. 13), inflammatory arthritis (p. 12), gout, food intolerance (p. 11), circulatory problems (p. 12) or pain referred from the hip or lower back (p. 219). Reflex sympathetic dystrophy (p. 10) can affect the joint.

Ankle injuries

The bones and soft tissues of the ankle can be damaged through trauma or overuse at any age. Ankle injury always disrupts the proprioceptive balance mechanisms. It also has a direct effect on the foot and lower leg muscles, disrupts the rest of the leg on the same side, and usually causes overload on the opposite side.

Bone traumatic fracture

The bones around the ankle can be broken by severe twisting stress or vertical impact. This is an acute traumatic injury which can happen at any age. If the ankle joint is displaced, it is a fracture-dislocation. Damage to the bone's cartilage surface within the joint is called an osteochondral fracture. Injury to the talus, fibula or malleoli can cause cartilage or bone fragments to break off and form loose bodies in the ankle joint. Osteochondritis dissecans is a particular type of damage in a bone's cartilage surface, which happens especially in teenagers. In young children whose bones are still quite soft, fractures are termed 'greenstick'.

What you feel
A bone fracture can be surprisingly painless at first, and may seem no worse than a sprain. You may be able to put your weight on the foot. However, in a bad break there is acute pain, usually accompanied by swelling, bruising, perhaps bleeding, and visible deformity of the leg. Walking is painful or impossible. The ankle feels weak and becomes stiff. You may have throbbing pain at night or when you sit still. In the later stages you may notice a deep aching in the bones, which is a sign that they are healing.

Causes
A broken ankle can be caused by a fall, a wrench with the foot stuck in the ground, landing awkwardly from a jump, or a direct blow. Compression fractures happen more easily if your ankle is stiff or taped rigidly. You are more vulnerable to fracture if your bones are weakened by calcium deficiency, disease or osteoporosis.

Directions
You should receive immediate treatment in hospital. You may need surgery to stabilize the broken bones. Otherwise your leg may be immobilized in a plaster cast or a splint from the foot up to the knee or hip. In the early phase of healing, during the first ten days or so, the bones start the process leading to union, which normally happens after six to twelve weeks. Once the broken bone ends are joined together, the bones strengthen up and become slightly enlarged. Over the following months the damaged bones remodel themselves and gradually resume their normal shape.

How long?
9–18 months.

Ankle sprain

The soft tissues of the ankle can be torn, partly torn or overstretched as an acute traumatic injury which can happen at any age. If it is severe, there may also be bone damage which may not be obvious at first.

Types of sprain

In an *inversion sprain*, which is the most common, the foot and ankle turn inwards, and the lateral ligament takes the brunt of the force, sometimes cracking the fibula, and occasionally the medial malleolus too. In an *eversion sprain* the ankle twists outwards, straining the medial ligament, with damage to the medial malleolus and fibula in severe cases. In a *dorsiflexion sprain* the foot is forced upwards, compressing the structures at the front of the ankle, sometimes also causing damage to the talus and the soft tissues at the back of the ankle. In a *plantarflexion sprain* the foot is forced downwards, and the soft tissues on the top of the ankle are strained, while those behind the ankle are compressed.

What you feel

When the injury happens, there may be a lot of pain, or very little. Pain and stiffness may come on later. You may still be able to walk, or at least hobble, putting your foot down. With your foot off the ground, you can usually move the foot up and down, at least a little, but rotation is painful, difficult or impossible. Swelling may develop immediately or later. Bruising may appear around the joint straight away or later. A minor crack in any of the bones may cause localized swelling and tenderness if you press on it.

The amount of pain you feel does not necessarily reflect the degree of tissue damage. If a ligament is completely torn, there may be surprisingly little pain, but the ankle feels unstable and tends to give way if you try to put weight through the foot.

Causes

Ankle sprain can be caused by putting your foot down awkwardly, stepping on a ball or stone, catching your foot in a hole, tripping over the edge of a step or an opponent's foot, or using sports shoes which do not fit properly, or which have too much or too little grip for the playing surface. Ankle sprain happens more easily if you have stiff feet, knees or hips, or have suffered previous sprains or leg injuries which have created imbalance in the leg muscles and impaired your balance mechanisms.

Directions

For the first few days you may need an ankle support or firm bandaging and crutches. You should try to do frequent short walks taking a little weight through your foot.

How long?

2 weeks to 4 months.

Weak ankle

If the ankle ligaments have been badly torn, sometimes the ankle remains unstable after the initial pain and other symptoms have eased. There is a major loss of proprioception. Any of the ankle ligaments can be involved, including the inferior tibiofibular ligament and the retinacula which hold the ankle tendons in place. This is a chronic (long-standing) situation, and can happen at any age. In some cases an ankle can feel weak because of a stress fracture at the lower end of the fibula (see p. 93). Some people are born with abnormally weak ankles which tend to strain easily.

What you feel
The ankle is usually painless and functions adequately for normal activities. However, it tends to give way on uneven ground or when you play sports involving running, twisting and turning. When it gives way there may be pain and swelling.

Directions
You can use a stirrup splint for sports or walking on uneven ground. Avoid rigid taping or a tight sleeve support. Daily balance and strengthening exercises are essential. If the joint is very unstable, you may be advised to have surgery.

How long?
This is a long-term problem.

Chronic swelling

After recovery from an injury to your ankle or lower leg, the ankle may continue to swell. The fluid pools under the effect of gravity, so is usually minimal in the morning after a night's sleep, but worst in the evening, especially after sitting still for some time. It may also swell up after exercise involving running or jumping. In females hormonal changes linked to the menstrual cycle or pregnancy can make the swelling worse. Gravitational swelling is usually painless, although the feeling of puffiness may be unpleasant. If you do not control the swelling, it can affect the foot too.

Directions
Soft bandaging can help control the swelling. In some cases you may be advised to use support stockings. Avoid taping, tight ankle supports, boots and high-heeled shoes. Limit your activities to the amount which does not provoke a reaction, and check your diet, in case food intolerance is a factor (p. 11). If in doubt, refer to your doctor or specialist.

How long?
Several months.

Osteoarthritis (osteoarthrosis)

Wear-and-tear degeneration can happen in the ankle. It involves damage to the joint surfaces, loss of the normal space between the bones, and inflammation in the soft tissues. It usually occurs from late middle age onwards, although it can happen in younger people.

What you feel
The joint becomes stiff, but not necessarily painful. If pain occurs, it is often worst at night, or after weight-bearing activities such as walking, running or jumping. There may be swelling in the joint after exercise or in hot weather. You may notice increased pain when the weather changes, especially if rain is due. Sometimes there is thickening of the tissues around the ankle, making the ankle look permanently puffy. The ankle may be unusually hot or cool at times, and may tend to change colour, becoming redder or paler. The amount of pain you feel does not necessarily reflect the degree of arthritic damage in the joint. You might suffer surprisingly little pain despite an X-ray showing extensive damage, and vice versa.

Causes
Most often osteoarthritis is the long-term effect of previous injuries, such as repeated ankle sprains or a bad bone fracture close to the joint, especially if you restarted sport too soon after an injury. Sometimes it is the result of too much strenuous weight-bearing exercise, such as ultra-distance running. Some people have a hereditary tendency to the condition.

Directions
Use flexible, supportive shoes and cushioning insoles. Orthotics may help. Do daily exercises to maintain strength and mobility in the joint. If you let the joint stiffen, the muscles around it weaken, and the problem gets progressively worse. Avoid taping and rigid supports. The fitter you are, the less osteoarthritis will interfere with your activities. If it causes you severe problems, you may be offered injections or surgery.

How long?
This is a long-term process.

Rehabilitation and recovery

Acute phase
Use the circulatory care measures (p. 27) and crutches according to your practitioner's instructions. Alternative training for the unaffected parts of your body should start as soon as possible (p. 25).

Early phase
As soon as you can move your ankle, you should start doing non-weight-bearing and isometric ankle exercises, combined with foot strengthening and mobilizing exercises (p. 56) and early stage walking exercises (p. 34), as your practitioner advises. The exercises are best done barefoot, if possible, but can also be done in soft flexible shoes. Add weights or a resistance for the strengthening exercises when possible. Aim at two or three sessions daily.

Recovery phase
When you can put your foot to the floor comfortably, you must do balance exercises (p. 36), as well as advanced exercises for correct walking (p. 38). Within pain limits, you should also do weight-bearing, stretching and advanced strengthening exercises for the calf (pp. 81–82), front thigh (pp. 126–128), hamstrings (pp. 135–137), inner thigh (pp. 144–146) and hip (pp. 162–166). Before going on to the final recovery phase (p. 308), you need to recover strength, especially soleus efficiency (p. 82, exercise 4), balance, and full mobility in the joint.

Re-injury prevention
After an injury, you may need to use a splint or stirrup taping to protect the ankle for certain activities, but do not tape the ankle rigidly in order to do sports which would otherwise cause pain. Balance exercises should be continued in the long term.

Basic dynamic ankle exercises

1. Sitting on the edge of a chair, or lying on your back, with your legs straight in front of you and heels on the floor, point both your feet downwards and upwards, as far as you comfortably can. 5–20 times. Repeat, moving the feet alternately.

2. Sitting on a chair with your legs straight, feet off the floor, point your feet downwards and upwards. 5–20 times both feet together, then repeat moving the feet alternately.

3. Sitting or lying on the floor with your legs straight in front of you, feet apart, turn your feet inwards so that the soles face each other, then turn them outwards. 5–20 times.

4. Sitting or lying down with your legs straight in front of you, feet apart, make circles with your feet, first with both moving in the same direction, then in opposite directions. 5–20 times.

5. Sitting on a chair with your knees bent and feet flat, lift your toes and foot upwards at the ankle, then slowly lower them downwards. 5–10 times.

6. As exercise 5, but sit on a raised support so that your foot is off the floor. 5–10 times.

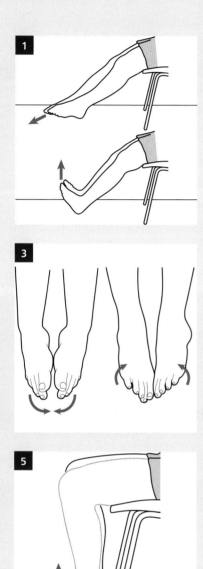

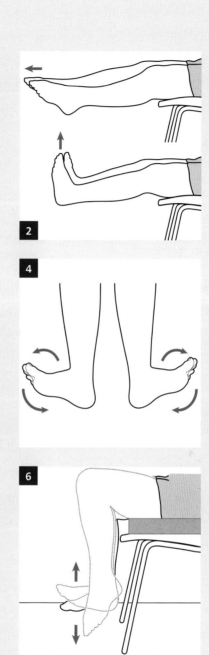

Isometric ankle strengthening exercises

1. Sitting or lying down, place one foot on top of the other; tense the lower foot as if to lift it into dorsiflexion, and press the sole of the upper foot down against the lower foot for a count of 5, resisting any movement, then relax completely. Reverse the position of the feet and repeat. 3–6 times.

2. Sitting with your knees bent or straight, or lying on your back with your legs straight, cross your ankles so that the outer edges of your feet touch; press the outer edges of your feet together for a count of 5, then relax completely. 3–6 times.

3. Sitting or lying on your back with your legs straight, turn your feet inwards so that the inner edges touch; press the inner edges of your feet together for a count of 5, then relax completely. 3–6 times.

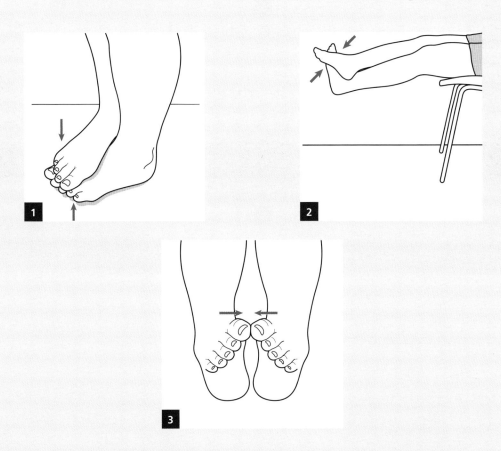

Chapter 6

The Calf Muscles
and Achilles Tendon

RIGHT CALF AND ACHILLES TENDON, SEEN FROM BEHIND.

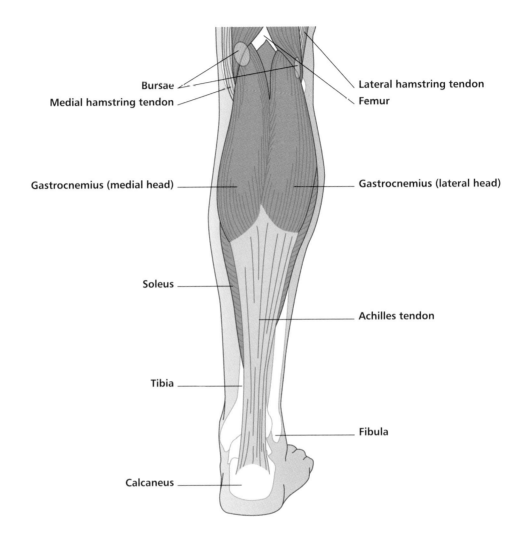

Gastrocnemius, soleus and plantaris are the calf muscles, which, together with the Achilles tendon, lie on the back of the lower leg between your knee and your heel.

Structure

Gastrocnemius forms the bulky part at the upper end of the lower leg. It has two parts, the lateral and medial heads, on the outer and inner sides of the leg respectively. From two tendons just above the back of the knee gastrocnemius extends down to merge with the Achilles tendon. Underlying gastrocnemius is soleus, which is attached to the back of the tibia and fibula, and also merges with the Achilles tendon. You can feel and see soleus on either side of the tendon, low down in the leg.

The Achilles tendon stands out as the thickest and strongest tendon in the body. At its lower end, just above its attachment point on the calcaneus, the tendon becomes thinner and more rounded. There is a kind of triangular 'space' behind the ankle between the lower end of the tendon and the underlying structures. Because the tendon is not close to any friction-causing structures, it does not have a fluid-filled synovial sheath, but is covered with a fibrous lining called a paratenon. At this lower end of the tendon the blood supply is very poor, and this was the famous weak point of the Greek warrior Achilles. A bursa, or small sac, of fluid separates the tendon from the upper part of the calcaneus, to allow friction-free movement.

Plantaris is a thin muscle on the back of the calf between gastrocnemius and soleus, which links into the medial (inner) edge of the Achilles tendon. These muscles cover the deep-lying posterior tibial muscles (p. 86) and popliteus (p. 86).

What they do

The calf muscles and Achilles tendon are active when you walk, run, jump and hop. When they contract and shorten they bend the ankle so that the foot points downwards into plantarflexion, allowing you to stand on tiptoe. Gastrocnemius also acts on the knee joint, helping the hamstrings to bend it.

Gastrocnemius is a fast-twitch muscle, and is especially well developed in people who run fast or jump a lot, such as sprinters, footballers, hockey players and ballet dancers. Soleus is a slow-twitch postural muscle which plays an important part in balance, especially when you stand on one leg. As the line of gravity falls slightly in front of the ankle when you stand still, soleus is in a constant state of slight tension to hold the upright position. Soleus is the prime mover when you go up and down on your toes keeping your knee locked straight: if soleus is weak, it is difficult to stop the knee from bending.

The Achilles tendon stores elastic energy, releasing it as needed for momentum and shock absorption. If the tendon lengthens for any reason, it loses tension, reducing your ability to spring and sprint. Rowers used to have lengthened Achilles tendons when rowing boats had footplates which held the feet fixed, so aerobic land training was better done on bicycles. Now that footplates allow mobility, oarsmen can run efficiently.

The calf muscles help the body's circulatory flow. Unlike the arteries which deliver oxygenated blood round the body, the veins which transport the blood back from the foot towards the heart for re-oxygenation do not contain active muscles. The blood is pushed up through the veins as the leg muscles contract – a system known as the 'muscle pump'. Valves in the veins prevent the blood from flowing in the wrong direction as the muscles relax.

If your hamstrings are weak for any reason, gastrocnemius compensates by generating extra strength when you bend your knee against a resistance. If gastrocnemius and soleus are both weakened, the deep posterior tibial muscles compensate when you try to point your foot downwards. This makes your toes curl, for instance if you stand on tiptoe.

Pain and complications

Gradual or unexplained pain and swelling in your calf can be caused or aggravated by circulatory problems (p. 12). Intermittent claudication is a condition in which the leg arteries become deficient, causing severe, pulsating pain. Thrombosis (a blood clot) in a vein can cause a localized point of strong pain and tenderness. Reflex sympathetic dystrophy (p. 10) can give rise to severe pain and disability following a seemingly trivial injury.

Pain can also be referred to the calf region from the back or hip. Hip problems can cause pain in the lower end of the Achilles tendon. Cramping pain in the calves can be due to dehydration, mineral deficiency, certain illnesses, some medicines, and, in some cases, performance-enhancing drugs. Calf muscle discomfort can also be a symptom of a stress fracture in one of the leg bones.

Calf cramp

Sudden spasm in the calf muscles is a common problem in sporting and non-sporting people alike, at any age. It can happen during activity, rest or sleep. Severe leg cramp after sport is sometimes called a 'charley horse'.

What you feel
The effects of calf cramp range from a mild tension in the muscles to severe tightness and agonizing pain.

Causes
Because of their close association with the circulatory system, the lower leg muscles reflect any adverse changes in the blood flow. Calf cramps, especially at night, happen most often because of dehydration, sometimes combined with overexercising. In very hot humid climates, loss of minerals can be a factor. Females can become prone to calf cramps related to the menstrual cycle or pregnancy, and are more vulnerable if they are dehydrated or mineral-deficient. Other contributory factors include stress, raised cholesterol, varicose veins and certain medicines. Soleus muscle strain can cause cramping in the calf, especially when you walk or try to run.

Directions
Calf cramps are usually eased by moving the foot and leg, gently stretching the calves, walking around and drinking water. In a humid climate or hot conditions you may also need to take in more minerals, including salt. If you suffer cramps often, and are not sure why, you should consult your doctor.

Restless legs syndrome

Discomfort in the calf area of the legs at rest, especially in bed, is a disturbing problem which affects a lot of people, mainly adults, including sports players. Some people have the symptoms mainly during the evening and night, others during the day as well. The problem can be intermittent. If recurrent, it tends to get worse as you get older.

What you feel
There may be tingling, itching, numbness, pain or an electrical sensation. Your legs feel as though they need to move. Symptoms can be relieved, at least partially, by weight-bearing exercises or walking around.

Causes
Dehydration, poor diet, and iron and magnesium deficiency can be factors. In females the problem can be linked to pregnancy or menstruation. Various conditions are also associated with the problem, including peripheral neuropathy (malfunction in the legs' nerve systems), thyroid problems, diabetes, coeliac disease and rheumatoid arthritis.

Directions
Try improving your water and food intake, especially by cutting down or avoiding irritants like alcohol, caffeine, fizzy drinks and refined sugar. If the problem becomes long-standing, you should refer to your doctor.

Varicose veins

Two sets of veins, *deep* and *superficial*, take blood back towards the heart from the foot. Congestion can happen if the valves controlling the blood flow become faulty, allowing pooling to occur. The superficial veins close to the skin become more prominent, enlarged and twisted, sometimes causing pain. At worst the veins can become fragile and bleed easily, causing bruising under the skin or external bleeding if the skin is thin.

Causes
Varicose veins can be hereditary. They happen when your blood flow has been impaired for any reason. Sitting or standing still for long periods, insufficient exercise, obesity, frequent air travel and hormone changes due to pregnancy can be contributory factors. They can also appear after an injury in any part of the leg. Although they may become apparent during teenage years, varicose veins are most common in adults, especially in later life.

Directions
If the problem is not severe, varicose veins can be controlled through exercise, support stockings, gentle massage with arnica or heparinoid cream (p. 29), and avoiding adverse pressure on the legs. If the veins become painful and tend to burst, they should be assessed by a vascular surgeon, who can offer an appropriate choice of treatments, usually either injection or surgery. Exercise is recommended after treatment.

Calf muscle and Achilles tendon injuries

The calf muscles and Achilles tendon can be injured through trauma or overuse at any age. Shoes are often a factor. Trauma can involve external factors, but is often intrinsic.

Injury has a direct effect on the foot, ankle, knee and hip joints, and the leg muscles, especially the hamstrings, on the same side, and can cause overload on the opposite leg.

Achilles tendon insertion strain

The tendon can be strained or suffer a minor tear at its attachment to the calcaneus. Sometimes the bursa between the tendon and the upper part of the bone becomes inflamed. In a chronic problem, spurs may form on the calcaneus. A spur can become detached, forming a focal point of pain. Achilles insertion problems can occur at any age. In children it is often linked to Sever's 'disease' (p. 51).

What you feel
Pain usually comes on gradually, although it can happen suddenly. You feel pain on tiptoeing or running. The heel is tender when you press on it. In the early stages the pain may wear off when you are warmed up, but recurs later during your exercise. The tendon gradually tightens. There is little or no pain at rest unless there is direct pressure on the heel.

Causes
There is usually excessive strain on the calf in extreme ranges of movement, for instance when you run uphill as fast as you can. Shoes contribute if they have rough, uneven linings round the heel; if the heel counter is soft, tight or not the right shape for your foot; if the sole is hard; or if the heel has worn down unevenly.

Directions
Check your shoes and discard any which chafe, if padding does not help. You may benefit from orthotics. Your doctor or specialist may offer you an injection.

How long?
Up to several months.

Achilles tendon injury, just above the heel

The tendon can become sore, thickened and tender to touch at the back of the ankle or just above, on one or both legs. The condition is called Achilles peritendinitis, meaning inflammation in the paratenon. It is an overuse problem which happens mainly to teenagers and adults, but can happen even to very young children.

What you feel
Symptoms may appear gradually or suddenly. You feel pain during sport. First thing in the morning there is stiffness in the tendon, which wears off as you move around. There is no

pain at rest. The tendon might hurt if you go up and down on your toes barefoot, but in the early stages this pain eases with repetitions. Going up and down on your toes wearing shoes usually causes pain. In the later stages, the tendon hurts when you walk and when there is any kind of pressure against it, for instance if you sit with your ankles crossed.

Causes

If you feel the pain when you wear certain shoes, but not barefoot, the cause is friction from the back of the shoe. Most sports shoes have raised backs, known as heel tabs, as do many normal shoes. It may look low, but if the tab is any higher than the level of the ankle it puts pressure on the Achilles tendon. Boots with stiff seams do the same. Once the problem starts, any shoes which touch the Achilles tendon make it worse.

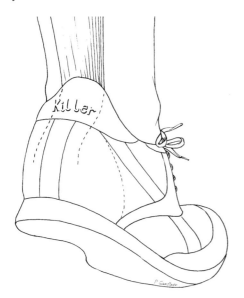

A high heel tab presses on the Achilles tendon, or can irritate the Achilles tendon.

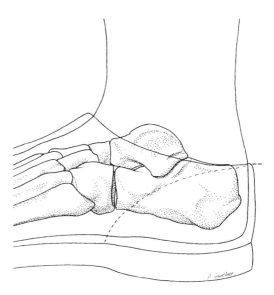

The shoe back should be no higher than the heel bone.

Other causes or aggravating factors of this type of pain include overtraining; faulty foot mechanics, especially overpronation; pain referred from the hip; poor circulation caused by sitting too long in tight clothing or with your ankles crossed; and hormonal changes in females.

Directions

Any faulty shoes must be discarded or modified by cutting the heel tabs back to the right level. In some cases this solves the problem immediately.

Some specialists offer injections into the painful tendon: if you choose this option, make sure your specialist is an expert, otherwise there is a strong risk of tendon rupture a few weeks later. A more drastic option in chronic cases is surgery to strip the tendon clean of inflammatory material.

How long?

3 days to 6 months.

The Calf Muscles and Achilles Tendon

Achilles tendon rupture

A total tear in the Achilles tendon can happen in any part of its length. It is a sudden, traumatic injury. When the tendon snaps, it leaves two broken ends which may stay close together or spring apart, leaving a visible dent. There may also be bruising and swelling.

Rupture is very rare in children, uncommon in teenagers, and happens most often to people in early and later middle age.

What you feel
You feel as if something has hit you hard in the back of the leg. If you try to walk, you stumble or fall over. Your foot feels floppy: you can draw the foot upwards into dorsiflexion, but while the toes can still move downwards into flexion, you cannot point the foot down at the ankle. If you lie on your stomach, the foot falls to a right angle. If the gastrocnemius muscle is squeezed, the foot does not move as it normally would: this is a standard test for Achilles tendon rupture, and does not cause pain.

Causes
Although the rupture can be caused by a direct blow to the back of the leg when the calf is under tension, more often it is intrinsic, with no obvious cause. It usually happens late in an exercise session or competition, and is associated with fatigue and circulatory problems rather than being cold or not warmed up properly. You may have had previous warning signs, such as tightness, cramping or involuntary twitching in the calf. You may have been stressed, overtired or suffering from an infection. The tendon may have been weakened by previous injury or injection, or overworked by compensating for a previous thigh or foot injury.

Directions
The foot must be supported immediately with bandaging or taping in the plantarflexed position, pointing down from the ankle. Avoid putting weight through it: hop using crutches or leaning on a helper. If you have to put the foot down, keep the leg away from your body turned out sideways, and try to keep your weight on the heel.

Seek specialist advice as quickly as possible. You have the choice of an operation or non-intervention. Surgery can be done through a scar as open surgery, or 'blind' (closed) through a series of holes in the skin. The latter is known as the 'Ma technique' after its inventor, and only very skilled surgeons perform it successfully.

Non-intervention is a choice between either immobilization in a plaster cast for several weeks, or support in a removable walking boot (pictured left) which allows weight-bearing, remedial therapies, exercises and alternative training to commence immediately. You should decide with your practitioner which approach you want to use, and then follow all instructions to the letter.

Rehabilitation phases
In all cases the foot is held pointing downwards in plantarflexion for the first phase, as the tendon has to be prevented from lengthening as it heals. If it is not in plaster, the leg can be taped to hold the position. Crutches are used as directed by the specialist. In the case of the walking boot they may not be needed for long, but should be used when exercises are done without the boot on.

Rehabilitation starts with calf strengthening holding the Achilles tendon in a shortened position. Progression through the rehabilitation phases should generally be pain-free. However, sometimes following open surgery there is a moment when some movement causes a tearing sensation around the scar, almost as if the injury has happened again. This is usually due to adhesions round the scar breaking, and does not interfere with your progress to fitness. If in doubt, refer back to your practitioner.

How long?
While functional recovery can be quicker, allow at least 9–12 months before returning to demanding or high-level sports.

Achilles tendon partial tear

A partial rupture of the Achilles tendon can feel as dramatic as a total tear, but you can still point your foot downwards, and squeezing the calf above the level of the injury produces downward movement of the foot.

Directions
Treatment and rehabilitation follow the same pattern as for a total rupture.

How long?
At least 3 months.

Calf muscle tear and strain

Any of the calf muscles can suffer a tear or strain, sometimes resulting in internal bleeding or bruising and muscle tightness. Gastrocnemius is injured most often, while soleus is rarely damaged on its own. Most often the injury is sudden and traumatic, but the calf muscles can also suffer from overuse damage. Tears and strains happen mainly to adults, less often to teenagers. More rarely, they can occur in children, sometimes in association with 'growing pains' (p. 87).

What you feel
In a traumatic injury there may be a feeling that something has 'snapped' or tightened up suddenly in a painful cramp. A tear in plantaris can feel just like an Achilles tendon rupture. The affected area feels painful to touch. It may show immediate bruising and sometimes also swelling. An overuse strain starts with slight pain or cramping felt during or after activity, which gradually gets worse if you continue.

The Calf Muscles and Achilles Tendon

Causes
The traumatic tear or strain can happen through overexertion in sports, sudden changes of direction while running or hopping, or overstretching because of an awkward movement or fall. Overuse injury is generally the result of overload through excessive repetitions of running or jumping drills, or because the calf muscles are compensating for a previous problem in the foot or hamstrings. Calf muscle injuries are more likely to happen if you are dehydrated or overtired. Some performance-enhancing supplements might play a part. Hormone changes related to the menstrual cycle or pregnancy can make females more vulnerable.

Directions
You should use a heel lift or shoes with heels in the first phase, to avoid irritation. You may need crutches for the first few days. Soft bandaging from your toes to just below the knee can help control swelling. Do not rub the muscles directly in the acute phase.

How long?
4 weeks to 4 months.

Gastrocnemius tendon injury

One or both of the gastrocnemius tendons may be damaged where they attach to the thigh bone behind the knee. There may be a tear in the tendon itself, or inflammation in the bursa under the tendon. Most often this is an overuse injury which comes on gradually, but sometimes it happens suddenly. Injury can happen at any age, but is uncommon in children.

What you feel
Usually there is a small focal point of pain behind the knee which is tender to touch. You feel pain if you exert the calf muscles strongly, for example when sprinting up stairs.

Causes
You can overstretch the tendons, for instance when doing a high kick in rugby or football, or by doing overenthusiastic hamstring and calf stretches. Injury can also happen through forced or prolonged twisting movements with the knee fully bent, as in limbo dancing.

Directions
Avoid painful activities, and try to maintain efficiency in the vastus medialis obliquus muscle (p. 112).

How long?
Despite being relatively minor, it can take 3 months or more.

Rehabilitation and recovery

Acute phase
Use the circulatory care measures (p. 27) according to your practitioner's instructions. You may need crutches at first (p. 32). Alternative training for the unaffected parts of your body should start as soon as possible (p. 25).

Early phase
After the acute phase, when your practitioner allows, you should start doing the basic calf and Achilles exercises. They are designed to strengthen the calf muscles and Achilles tendon with the tendon held at its optimum length, and are essential following total or partial Achilles tendon rupture and any major injury to the calf muscles. Aim at one to three sessions daily.

Recovery phase
When you can put your heel flat to the floor without discomfort, you should progress to the calf stretching exercises and the advanced strengthening exercises. They should be combined, as possible, with exercises to improve your walking pattern (p. 34) and balance (p. 36), and advanced strengthening exercises for the front thigh (p. 128), hamstrings (p. 137), inner thigh (p. 146) and hip (p. 166).

It is vital to regain soleus function (advanced calf strengthening, exercise 4) before starting the final recovery phase (p. 308).

The Calf Muscles and Achilles Tendon

Basic calf and Achilles strengthening exercises

1. Sitting on a chair, or standing using a support or crutches, put your toes and forefoot on a weighing scale, heel up; press your weight down through the ball of the foot, keeping your heel up and knee bent. 3–10 times. Work towards taking 80–90% of your body weight through the ball of the foot.

2. Sitting or lying down, practise pointing your foot downwards. As your calf muscles get stronger, try to keep the toes relaxed so that they do not curl downwards.

3. Sitting with your feet pointing downwards, toes on the floor and heels up, try to lift your heels a little more, then relax. 5–10 times, first with both feet together, then alternately.

4. Using crutches, wearing the walking boot or with taping, practise walking, taking some weight through the toes, without letting your heel go flat to the floor.

5. When you can take at least 50% of your body weight through the toes with your knee bent, practise with your knee straight: standing with your good leg on a support level with the weighing scale, place your injured leg with knee straight on the weighing scale, and press through the ball of the foot, keeping the heel up. 3–10 times.

6. When you can take 90% of your body weight through the ball of the foot, gradually practise bringing the heel down to the floor, in easy stages.

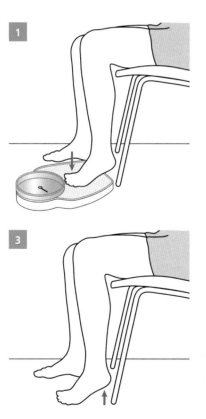

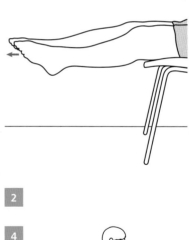

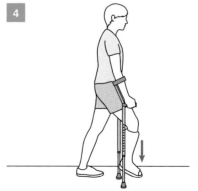

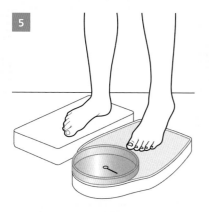

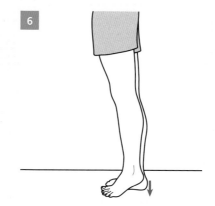

Calf and Achilles stretching

1. **Gastrocnemius stretch**. Standing with your legs parallel, feet pointing forwards, place your injured leg slightly behind you with your knee straight and heel flat on the floor. Hold the position for a count of 6, then relax completely. As flexibility improves, you can place the leg further back in easy stages. 3–10 times.

2. **Soleus stretch**. Standing with your legs parallel, feet pointing forwards, place your injured leg behind you and bend your knee until you feel a gentle stretching sensation along the lower calf; hold for a count of 6, then relax completely. 3–10 times.

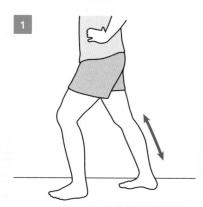

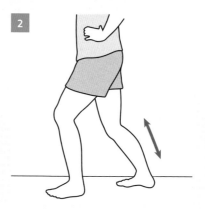

The Calf Muscles and Achilles Tendon

Advanced calf and Achilles strengthening exercises

1. **Calf raise**. Standing on two legs, go up and down on your toes, knees bent at first, then with knees straight. 5–20 times.

2. **Calf raise with weight transfer**. Standing with your legs apart and your knees straight, go up on your toes, shift your weight over your injured leg, then lower your heels with control, keeping your knees straight throughout. 5–20 times.

3. **Gastrocnemius strengthener**. Using a support if necessary, stand on your injured leg and go up and down on your toes, with your knee bent. Keep your toes as relaxed as possible. 3–10 times.

4. **Soleus strengthener**. Standing on your injured leg beside a support, go up and down on your toes, keeping your knee straight. Try to keep your toes as relaxed as possible. 3–10 times. Hold weights in your hands when the exercise becomes easy, starting light and building up in easy stages.

5. **Calf raise through range**. Standing with the ball of the foot of your injured leg on the edge of a step, drop your heel downwards with control, then go up on your toes, keeping your knee straight. 3–10 times.

6. **Complex calf raise**. Standing on your injured leg beside a support, bend your knee, keeping your foot flat on the floor; straighten the knee and go up on your toes keeping the knee locked straight; then bring the heel down and bend the knee again. This is a continuous cycle: build up from 3 movements to 10 without stopping.

7. **Up steps**. Using the handrail as necessary, walk up steps, pushing off the ball of the foot. 5 steps, building up to 10 or more. Gradually increase your speed.

8. **Down steps**. Using the handrail as necessary, walk down steps, keeping the foot as straight forward as possible, and using the ball of the foot. 2–3 steps, building up to 10 or more.

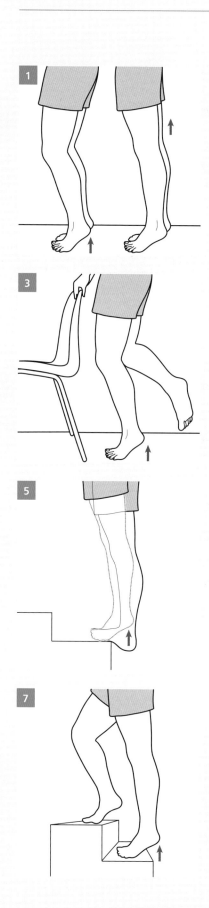
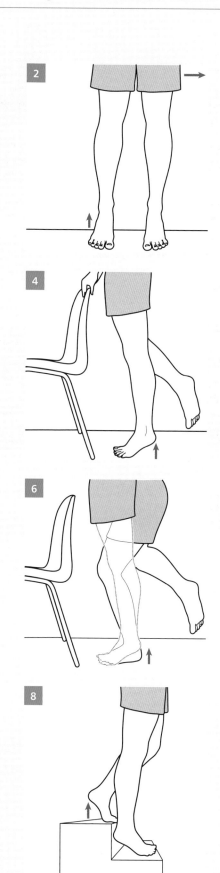

7

The Shin and Lower Leg

RIGHT LOWER LEG, SEEN FROM THE FRONT.

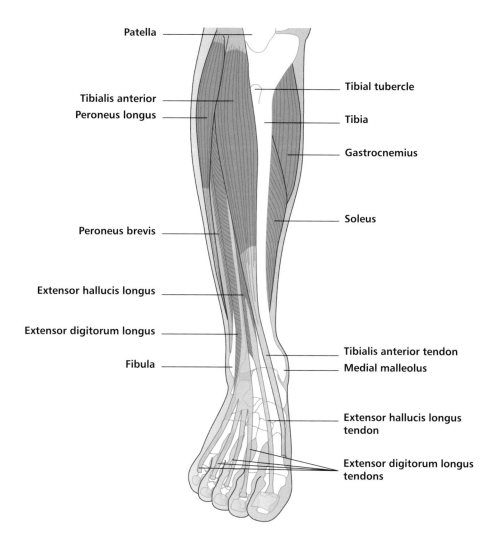

Patella

Tibialis anterior
Peroneus longus

Peroneus brevis

Extensor hallucis longus

Extensor digitorum longus

Fibula

Tibial tubercle

Tibia

Gastrocnemius

Soleus

Tibialis anterior tendon
Medial malleolus

Extensor hallucis longus
tendon

Extensor digitorum longus
tendons

The lower leg, which includes the shin, links the ankle and the knee.

Structure

It consists of two long bones linked by muscles and other soft tissues.

Bones

The tibia (shinbone) is the main weight-bearing bone linking the ankle to the knee. You can feel the flat edge of the bone along the front inner side of the lower leg, where it lies directly under the skin. In front at the top, just below the centre of the knee, it has a bony knob called the tibial tubercle or tuberosity. At its lower inner edge, the tibia ends in a protrusion, known as the medial malleolus, on the inner (medial) side of the ankle.

On the outer side of the lower leg is the fibula (outer leg bone), a slender non-weight-bearing bone which extends from the knee to the ankle. At its lower end it expands to form the lateral malleolus, which is visible on the outer side of the ankle. You can feel the head of the fibula just below the knee, but beyond that the bone is more difficult to feel as it is covered by the fleshy calf muscles.

Joints

The tibia and fibula are connected at the top and bottom by strong ligaments to form the superior (upper) and inferior (lower) tibiofibular joints. The upper joint is synovial, as it is bound within a fluid-filled capsule, whereas at the lower joint the bones are simply tied by ligaments in what is technically known as a syndesmosis. In between the two bones, almost down their whole length, is a strong band called the interosseous membrane, which creates a partition between the front and back of the lower leg.

Muscles

Long muscles extend from the leg bones down to the foot and toes. You can feel them working if you put your hand round your leg and move your toes.

Tibialis anterior forms the fleshy bulk over the front of the lower leg. It runs from the outer side of the upper part of the shinbone down to the medial cuneiform and the base of the first metatarsal in the foot. Extensor digitorum longus spreads mainly from the outer part of the top of the tibia and the inner part of the upper fibula down to the ends of the toes. Extensor hallucis longus runs from the inner side of the fibula and the interosseous membrane to the top of the end part of the big toe. The cords of the extensor tendons stand out on the top of your foot when you lift your toes off the floor.

On the back of the lower leg, flexor hallucis longus extends mainly from the fibula and interosseous membrane to the underside of the end of the big toe, while flexor digitorum longus follows a parallel path downwards from the back of the tibia to the other toes. Tibialis posterior lies underneath the flexors, and is attached to the back of the interosseous membrane and the upper parts of the tibia and fibula. It runs down behind the inner side of the ankle, fixes on to the navicular and the two cuneiforms next to it, and ends in attachments under the bases of the second to fourth metatarsals in the foot.

At the upper end of the tibia and fibula there are attachment points for various thigh muscles which act on the knee. The patellar tendon, the end point of quadriceps, is attached to the tibial tubercle. The hamstring tendons are attached behind the upper ends of the tibia and fibula. Popliteus is a small, flat muscle at the back of the knee, linking the femur and knee capsule to the back of the upper end of the tibia. At the outer side of the knee, the iliotibial tract attaches to the upper ends of the tibia and fibula.

Functions

You cannot move the two lower leg bones individually. They work in conjunction with the knee at their upper ends, and the ankle and foot below. There is a slight gliding movement between the upper ends of the tibia and fibula, which happens automatically when the knee moves, also, though minimally, during ankle movements. At its lower end, the fibula twists slightly outwards when the foot is drawn up at the ankle into dorsiflexion, enlarging the gap between the tibia and fibula to allow space for the wider front part of the talus.

Pain and complications

Unexpected or unexplained pain in the shin region can be caused by circulatory problems, infection, reflex sympathetic dystrophy (p. 10), pain referred from the hip or back, or, very rarely, bone disease or a tumour.

'Growing pains'

In children unexplained pain can occur anywhere in the legs, but often affects the lower legs, usually both at the same time. It happens sometimes in children as young as two, occasionally in teenagers, but mostly around five to seven years.

What you feel
The pain can be extremely severe. It tends to happen late in the day or at night. Relief is difficult to find.

Causes
The pain is not directly related to particular activities, although sometimes it comes on after hard running sessions. It can coincide with a growth spurt, but a link to growth has not been proved, despite the name. It can coincide with headaches and abdominal pain, so it might be linked to allergies. Dehydration is often a factor, and sometimes stress and overtiredness too.

Directions
There is no specific treatment. You have to check through the possible factors and try to eliminate them. Drinking enough water is especially important.

How long?
A few weeks, sometimes much longer.

Shin and lower leg injuries

The bones and soft tissues of the lower leg can be injured through trauma or overuse at any age. Injury disrupts function in the foot, ankle, knee, hip and lower back on the same side, and can cause overload on the opposite leg.

Tibial traumatic fracture

A break in the shinbone is a traumatic injury which can be across the bone, down its length, or diagonal, known as a horizontal, vertical or spiral fracture respectively. The injury can happen in conjunction with a bad twist to the ankle or knee, and can cause damage to nerves and blood vessels. It can happen at any age. In young children trauma to the shaft can cause a greenstick fracture, in which one side of the bone breaks while the other holds together but bends. Damage close to either end of the bone can disrupt the epiphysis (growth area).

What you feel

A major fracture which causes the bone to snap can be surprisingly painless at the time of the accident, although pain can build up over the next few hours. The leg swells. The skin may remain intact, or there might be an open wound. Active movement using the muscles round the fracture site is difficult or impossible. If the nerves are damaged, there may be numbness or tingling. Shock can set in following the accident.

A more minor break which leaves the bone in line, without skin damage, can be very painful, but the other symptoms are less dramatic. It is usually still possible to move the foot and knee, albeit with pain. Putting full weight on the foot is not possible.

As the bone heals you may feel a deep aching in it, which is normal, provided there are no other symptoms. After about six weeks, you may notice that the area around the fracture looks enlarged, and this is a sign of bone proliferation, which is part of the mending process. Usually the enlarged area reduces over time, but sometimes the leg stays slightly deformed compared to the other leg.

Causes

As the tibia is a strong weight-bearing structure, it takes a violent impact or shearing force to break it, such as an awkward fall or a tackling foul, especially if the foot gets stuck as the impact happens. The bone will break more easily if it is diseased or osteoporotic, or if you suffer from mineral deficiency.

Directions

You have to be treated in hospital as an emergency. You may need an immediate operation to realign or stabilize the broken bone. Otherwise your leg may be immobilized in a plaster cast extending from your toes or your ankle to below your knee or sometimes up to your hip, according to the nature of the fracture. You will probably have to stay in bed for the first phase of healing, and use crutches when you are allowed up.

Complications such as infection, non-union or reflex sympathetic dystrophy (p. 10) delay the healing process. If warning signs appear, like unusual pain, hot swelling, skin discolouration or raised temperature, refer back to your practitioner immediately.

How long?
9–18 months.

Shinbone bruise

The front edge of the tibia is especially vulnerable to bone bruising, as it lies under the skin without any protective muscle padding. Trauma can cause bleeding between the bone and its covering, or periosteum. A swollen lump forms over the surface of the bone, technically called a subperiosteal haematoma. It is a traumatic injury which can happen at any age.

What you feel

The injury causes immediate pain, followed by swelling and bruising. The damaged area may feel slightly numb. If you prod it, it feels tender.

Causes
The damage is caused by a direct blow, kick or knock.

Directions
Ice or a cold compress should be applied immediately (p. 29), and the lower leg should be bandaged with soft compressive material from the toes to below the knee. In a severe injury you may need to go to hospital to check whether the shinbone has been broken. You can apply gentle massage with arnica or heparinoid cream around the haematoma, but you should avoid pressing directly over it.

As the haematoma reduces in size and becomes less painful, you can gradually resume your normal activities. Protect the shinbone from direct knocks with shin guards or padded bandaging.

How long?
3–12 weeks, sometimes longer.

Tibial stress fracture

The shinbone can develop cracks through overstrain. Stress fractures can happen in any part of the bone, at any age, but are least common in children.

What you feel
Pain starts gradually. The first sign is usually after training or at night. If you keep doing the same type of exercise, the pain gets progressively worse. It can even get to the stage where you have pain when walking, although you can still do other activities involving the legs, such as cycling, without pain. You may feel tenderness if you press on the affected area of the bone. In some cases you may notice redness or slight swelling over the painful area.

Causes
A stress fracture is caused by repetitive muscle pull against the bone, which is more than normal. It means you are doing too much, too often. Jarring stresses are not the main cause, so running on soft surfaces does not prevent stress fractures. The problem is always linked to a change in activities: you may have started doing running training from scratch or after a lay-off, increased your training mileage, or taken up skipping for fitness. If you space out your repetitive training, your bones will adapt and strengthen, so they will not crack, but if you do sessions without allowing enough recovery time, the hard surface of the bone starts to break down. Stress fractures happen in healthy bones, but occur more easily if a bone is weakened by mineral deficiency or osteoporosis.

Directions
As a stress fracture usually does not show up on X-ray until it is healing, it is diagnosed on the basis of your description of your pain and activities, and if necessary a bone scan. You must rest from running and repetitive training for eight weeks or longer, according to your practitioner's advice. Pain-free alternative training and exercises will help the crack to heal. Avoid 'trying out' the leg before it heals, as you risk prolonging the problem. At worst, the bone crack can develop into a complete fracture.

How long?
4–6 months.

'Shin soreness' and 'shin splints'

Pain over the front and sides of the shinbone is often described as 'shin soreness' or 'shin splints'. It is an overuse injury which becomes noticeable gradually. In some cases the pain comes on suddenly, but usually only after warning signs of discomfort. The problem might be a soft tissue strain affecting the tendons or muscles alongside the tibia, but very often it is a stress fracture. It can happen at any age, and is especially common in teenagers and young adults.

What you feel
Pain develops in the lower leg in stages, usually after exercise, especially running or walking long distances. If you continue with the same type of exercise, the pain gets worse, and eventually forces you to stop. It may get better after a few days' rest, but recurs quickly if you try the same exercise again. The pain may spread over the shin, or concentrate in a small area. There may be no tenderness at first when you press on the painful area, but later it becomes sore to touch. There may be pain when you do certain movements with the leg, or if you activate the muscles on either side of the shin against a resistance.

Causes
The most common cause is doing too much repetitive leg activity, such as running, walking, jumping, skipping or hopping. You may have just started an exercise programme, increased what you have been doing, or done sessions of repetitive training on a daily basis. Sometimes faulty foot mechanics or inappropriate shoes contribute. Occasionally the pain arises following tibial trauma, such as a kick. Poor circulation can be a factor.

Directions
The pattern of recovery is usually similar to that for a stress fracture.

How long?
2–6 months.

Shin muscle injury

Any of the muscles in the lower leg can be torn or strained at any age through trauma or overuse. Muscle injury can be complicated by circulatory problems, stress fracture or compartment syndrome.

What you feel
In an acute traumatic injury you feel immediate pain, sometimes together with a tearing feeling or sound. In an overuse injury pain comes on gradually in association with your activities. The injured area is tender if you press on it. You may notice slight swelling, wasting or bruising. The muscles hurt when they are active or stretched. If tibialis anterior is injured, for instance, it hurts to lift your foot upwards at the ankle, or to point your foot downwards, stretching the muscle. If the posterior tibial muscles are injured, it is painful when you contract them to point the toes and foot downwards and turn the foot inwards, or when you stretch them by drawing the foot upwards.

Causes

Traumatic tibial muscle injury can be part of a bad ankle sprain. A strain or tear can happen through a direct blow, or if you trip while the muscles are contracting. Overuse injury is most often caused by running or jumping too much on hard surfaces, especially if you have been trying to push off your toes more forcefully. Faulty foot mechanics and stiff or worn shoes can contribute. Sometimes circulatory problems play a part.

Directions

Check your shoes and discard any which are unsuitable. If foot mechanics have played a part, you may benefit from custom-fitted orthotics.

How long?

2–12 weeks.

Compartment syndrome

Excess fluid gathers and gets trapped inside an enclosing muscle sheath, causing tense swelling. When it affects the muscles on the front of the shin, it is called anterior tibial compartment syndrome, while at the back of the shin it is posterior tibial compartment syndrome. It is usually an overuse injury, but can happen through trauma. It can occur at any age, but is least common in children.

What you feel

In traumatic compartment syndrome the pain and swelling can happen quickly, and you may also have numbness and even loss of movement.

In an overuse injury the pain is usually associated with repetitive activities involving the legs, particularly running. It comes on when you exercise, starting with slight pain which becomes increasingly severe. The pain quickly eases off immediately after you stop the exercise, especially if you apply ice to the painful area (p. 29). However, if you continue, the pain starts to interfere with normal walking.

Sometimes compartment syndrome is complicated by an underlying stress fracture or a 'dropped foot' (p. 94) caused by nerve disruption.

Causes

Trauma can be caused by a direct blow. Overuse injury can happen if you have increased your training, changed from doing slow-paced running to sprinting, or started doing sessions of repetitive hopping or bounding. Changing your running pattern or foot biomechanics can be factors, as can using stiff or worn shoes. The problem is more likely to happen if your muscles are weak to start with.

Directions

A severe traumatic injury is treated as an emergency, because of the risk of circulatory complications. You have to avoid increasing the pressure on the leg, so you should not use tight bandaging or taping. Depending on the degree of damage, you may need an operation, called fasciotomy or decompression surgery, to release the tight sheath.

The initial phases of recovery usually involve doing slow movements to improve the deep-lying postural muscles in the calf and increase the circulatory flow. In some cases your therapist might use low-pulse electrical muscle stimulation (p. 20) to help the process. An overuse problem can become severe. If so, your practitioner will check that there are no circulatory complications or bone injuries. You may undergo pressure tests to identify whether there are significant changes in muscle pressure during and after exercise, compared to before exercise. If there are, you may be advised to have surgery.

How long?
3–12 weeks or more.

Tibial tubercle injury

Injury to the tibial tubercle always involves the patellar tendon. The tibial tubercle can be pulled away from the tibia by a sudden force in an avulsion fracture. It can also be cracked or bruised by a direct knock. Overstress through the patellar tendon can damage the tubercle: this is similar to a stress fracture. These injuries can happen at any age. In children and teenagers stress injury to the tibial tubercle, technically an apophysitis, is known as Osgood-Schlatter's condition, which happens most often between the ages of 11 and 14.

What you feel
If the tibial tubercle is separated completely or partially from the tibia through trauma, you cannot activate the quadriceps. The knee may look deformed, as the kneecap is no longer anchored properly. There may be little or lots of pain at first. A blow to the tibial tubercle is less disabling, and causes pain, bruising, swelling and movement inhibition.

Overuse injury causes gradually increasing pain on movements like going down stairs, squatting and kicking. There may also be pain sitting still. The pain eases with rest, but recurs if sports such as football, running or squash are resumed too soon. If you keep trying the leg out before it has healed, you risk getting an avulsion fracture.

Causes
Traumatic avulsion injury can be caused if the leg is blocked as the patellar tendon and quadriceps contract forcefully. The tubercle can be hit by a boot in rugby or a stick in hockey.

Overuse injury is caused by too much repetitive knee-bending activity, especially in sports like soccer, distance running, bowls, fencing and squash.

Directions
A severe avulsion fracture should be treated in hospital as quickly as possible. You may need surgery to fix the bone in the right position. For overuse injury to the tibial tubercle you must rest from painful or repetitive activities involving the knee until the area has healed. Do alternative training to help healing. As the pain subsides you should do gentle exercises to restore strength and flexibility around the knee.

How long?
Avulsion: 4–12 months.
Bruised tubercle: 4–8 weeks.
Overuse strain: 6–12 weeks.

Fibular traumatic fracture

The fibula can crack or break anywhere along its length at any age. It can break crosswise, lengthwise or spirally. Fracture at the upper end can happen together with damage to the knee or tibia, while at the lower end it can accompany ankle sprain. In young children trauma can cause greenstick fractures or damage to the epiphyses.

What you feel
Pain varies, and can build up over a few hours after the accident. There is usually swelling and sometimes also bleeding. The bone feels tender if you press it, and may look deformed. As it mends, you may feel a deep ache in the bone, and there may be an enlarged lump over the fracture site, which gradually reduces.

Causes
Fracture can be caused by a severe twisting strain, a direct blow, or a crush injury, if you fall sideways or your leg is trapped. The bone breaks more easily if you suffer from mineral deficiency or a bone condition such as osteoporosis.

Directions
If the bone is displaced, you should be treated in hospital as soon as possible. You may need an operation to realign the bone and fix the broken ends in position. Otherwise your leg may be immobilized in a plaster cast or a splint, which usually extends from the toes to below the knee. You will need to use crutches at first. As the fibula is not a weight-bearing bone, you may be allowed to put your foot to the floor at an early stage.

How long?
4–8 months.

Fibular stress fracture

The fibula can crack due to overuse injury. This can happen in any part of the bone, but is most common at the 'waist', the narrow part just above the ankle. It can occur at any age, but is rare in children.

What you feel
There is gradually increasing pain in the bone, usually after exercise at first, then during it. Pressure on the bone hurts. Most often there is no pain at rest. There may be redness or slight swelling over the painful area. If the fracture is at the lower end of the bone, there may be a feeling of weakness in the ankle.

Causes
Too much or a sudden build-up of repetitive activity causes pressure on the bone due to excessive muscle action. Faulty foot mechanics or poor shoes can contribute. Stress fractures happen in healthy bones, but are more likely if a bone is weakened by mineral deficiency or osteoporosis.

Directions

Diagnosis is made on the basis of your description of your pain pattern and your activities. You need to rest from painful and repetitive activities involving the leg until the bone heals. Avoid 'trying out' the leg before that, as you risk prolonging the problem, and the bone might break completely. Do painless alternative training and exercises to help promote the healing. Check your shoes and discard any which are worn or stiff. If your foot mechanics were part of the problem, you may benefit from custom-fitted orthotics. Allow two weeks after the bone has healed before gradually resuming your sport.

How long?
8–12 weeks.

'Dropped foot'

When you cannot lift your foot upwards at the ankle due to a kind of paralysis, it is known as 'dropped foot' or 'drop foot'.

What you feel
There may be tingling, numbness or a 'dead' feeling in the pathway of the damaged nerve down the lower leg. The foot feels floppy and drags as you walk.

Causes
A fracture, knock or prolonged pressure at the upper end of the fibula, just below the knee, can damage the peroneal nerve where it winds round the head of the bone. Sitting with your legs crossed can cause compression on the nerve. 'Dropped foot' can also be a complication of compartment syndrome, deep bruising or cuts in the anterior tibial muscles, total knee replacement surgery, a hip operation or 'trapped nerve' problems in the back (p. 219). Sometimes it is a sign of damage or disease in the central nervous system.

Directions
Your doctor will refer you for tests or to an appropriate specialist. You should wear well-fitting shoes: avoid any which increase the foot's tendency to drag. You may need to use a special splint to keep the foot in line.

How long?
Usually many months.

Rehabilitation and recovery

Acute phase

Use the circulatory care measures (p. 27) according to your practitioner's instructions. Alternative training for the unaffected parts of your body should start as soon as possible (p. 25).

Early phase

You need to regain function in all the muscles associated with the lower leg, so, depending on your situation, your initial programme may include foot strengthening, mobilizing and stretching exercises (p. 56); basic and isometric ankle exercises (pp. 66–68); basic calf strengthening (p. 80); essential vastus medialis obliquus (VMO) exercises (p. 112); and basic front-thigh (p. 127) and hamstring (p. 136) strengthening.

In a bone injury you become more active as the bone heals, allowing you to take more weight through the leg without pain. As soon as possible, your practitioner will recommend exercises such as the early stage exercises for correct walking (p. 34). Aim at two or three sessions a day.

Recovery phase

When you can take your full weight through the injured leg you should progress to doing the advanced exercises for correct walking (p. 38), the calf (p. 82), front thigh (p. 128) and hamstrings (p. 137), and you must work on your balance (p. 36). Before progressing to the final recovery phase (p. 308), you need to recover full mobility in the ankle and knee, plus strength and flexibility in all the leg muscle groups. Efficiency in soleus (exercise 4, p. 82) and good balance are essential.

8

The Knee

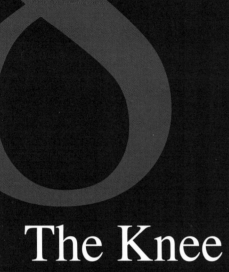

RIGHT KNEE SEEN FROM THE INNER (MEDIAL) SIDE.

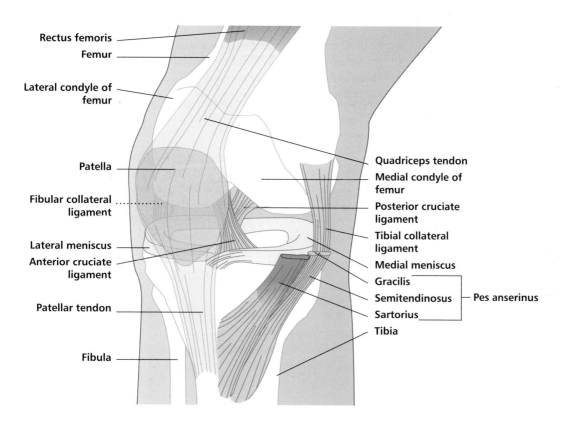

Rectus femoris
Femur
Lateral condyle of femur
Patella
Fibular collateral ligament
Lateral meniscus
Anterior cruciate ligament
Patellar tendon
Fibula

Quadriceps tendon
Medial condyle of femur
Posterior cruciate ligament
Tibial collateral ligament
Medial meniscus
Gracilis
Semitendinosus
Sartorius
Tibia
Pes anserinus

The knee is a compound joint linking the lower leg to the femur (thigh bone).

Structure

The knee consists of three parts: the tibiofemoral joint (or main knee joint), the patellofemoral joint and the superior tibiofemoral joint.

Bones and joints

The tibiofemoral joint is not a hinge but a condylar joint. The femoral condyles form a knuckle, roughly conforming to the two flattened, elliptical surfaces on top of the tibia.

The patellofemoral joint is a sellar (saddle) joint, formed where the small triangular patella, or kneecap, lies over the femur at the front of the knee. The patella is loosely held within the lower end of the quadriceps muscle, anchored by the patellar tendon.

The superior tibiofibular joint is a plane joint, formed between the top ends of the tibia and fibula (p. 86).

Capsule

The knee's capsule encloses the back and sides of the knee, and is attached to the sides of the kneecap, but does not cover the front. A fluid-forming synovial membrane lines the capsule and extends around the knee, reaching about five centimetres (two inches) above the kneecap. It lubricates the whole joint. Numerous bursae (fluid-filled pouches) lie between the tendons and ligaments around the knee, ensuring friction-free movement.

Ligaments

In the centre of the main knee joint are the two cruciate ligaments, which bind the femur to the tibia, and are called the anterior cruciate ligament (ACL) and the posterior cruciate ligament (PCL) according to their position on the tibia. The medial, or tibial, collateral ligament connects the femur and tibia on the inner side of the knee (facing the other leg). The lateral, or fibular, collateral ligament binds the outer side of the femur to the top of the fibula. The ligaments on the back of the knee are relatively weak. There is no ligament on the front of the knee. The patellar tendon is sometimes called the 'patellar ligament', although it is functionally a tendon.

Muscles and tendons

The quadriceps tendon attaches quadriceps femoris to the kneecap, while the patellar tendon is the end point of quadriceps and runs from the tip of the patella to the tibial tubercle. Under quadriceps lies the articularis genus, which is attached to the upper edge of the knee's synovial membrane. On the inner side of the knee, leading to the top of the tibia, are three tendons called the pes anserinus ('goose's foot'), which are the end points of sartorius, gracilis and semitendinosus. On the outer side of the knee there is a strong band called the iliotibial tract or iliotibial band, which links the hip muscles gluteus maximus and tensor fasciae latae to the top outer edges of the tibia and fibula. Behind the knee on either side are the prominent cords of the hamstring tendons, with the gastrocnemius tendons forming fleshy bulges between them. Popliteus (p. 86) lies more deeply behind the knee, where it is attached to the outer part of the femoral condyle, the joint capsule and the lateral meniscus.

Menisci (soft cartilages)

The knee's two menisci are also known as semilunar cartilages, because of their half-moon shape. They are attached to the top of the tibia by small ligaments. Their tips are called horns, with the anterior horns at the front of the knee and the posterior horns at the back. The medial meniscus, on the inner side, is elongated and attached to the medial ligament, while the lateral meniscus, on the outer side, is free-lying and more rounded. The menisci are lubricated by synovial fluid as the knee moves. Full lubrication of the posterior horns happens mainly when you squat down fully.

How the knee works

Because it combines freedom and stability, the knee allows for a wide variety of leg actions, such as running, jumping, kicking, dancing, skiing, kneeling and squatting. You can change direction nimbly and walk or run on uneven ground because of the way the knee coordinates with the foot, ankle, hip and pelvic joints.

Movements and muscles

The main muscles acting on the knee are quadriceps femoris over the front of the joint and the hamstrings at the back, helped by other muscles which coordinate with them. Quadriceps femoris straightens the knee against gravity, helped by the tensor fasciae latae acting through the iliotibial tract, and controls bending movements done under the influence of gravity, for instance when you walk down stairs or squat down slowly with control. If the knee is straightened against a very heavy load, the adductor muscles on the inside of the thigh join in, and the leg turns slightly inwards at the hip: this is a compensation mechanism. Articularis genus draws the pouch of synovial membrane above the front of the knee upwards as you straighten your knee.

The hamstrings bend the knee against gravity or a resistance, and control the reverse movement. They are helped by sartorius and gastrocnemius if necessary. Popliteus unlocks the knee when you start to bend it from the fully straight (hyperextended) position, and helps the posterior cruciate ligament to hold the femur steady when you crouch down. It may also act on the lateral meniscus, moving it when the knee is twisted outwards so that it is kept free from undue pressure between the bones.

The kneecap automatically glides up and down as the knee is bent and straightened. The only way to move the kneecap independently of the main knee joint is to contract quadriceps gently when the knee is straight. This is easier to do sitting down than standing up.

Because the condyles which form the lower end of the thigh bone are rounded and the medial condyle is slightly bigger than the other, the knee automatically twists outwards slightly as it straightens and inwards as it bends. Sitting with the knee bent to 90 degrees you can actively twist the knee inwards using the inner hamstrings and popliteus together with sartorius and gracilis, and outwards using the outer hamstring, biceps femoris. You can feel the hamstring cords working if you place your fingers over them as you do this.

Vastus medialis obliquus (VMO)

Vastus medialis is the inner part of the quadriceps group. At its lower end its fibres become more horizontal, forming vastus medialis obliquus (VMO), which is attached to the inner side of the kneecap, and is known as the 'key to the knee'. This small muscle is essential for locking the knee fully straight, controlling the kneecap from the inner side, and holding the kneecap steady in its groove between the femoral condyles. The VMO alone counteracts the influence of the other parts of quadriceps, which draw the kneecap outwards.

Knee variations

The shape of the knee is dictated by a lot of factors, including heredity, activities, muscle balance, the shape of the pelvis, postural habits, and the action of the ankles and feet. Flat, overpronated feet, in-turned hips or a widely spaced pelvis can contribute to 'knock-knee' (genu valgum), while a high-arched foot or a tendency to oversupinate, using the outer part of the foot, can contribute to 'bow leg' (genu varum). Bow legs can also be caused by encouraging a baby to stand up too early, before the bones and muscles are strong enough to take the weight. Excessive joint mobility can make the knee bend backwards when it is straightened into hyperextension. This is called genu recurvatum, and is often accompanied by patella alta, in which the kneecap sits higher than normal over the front of the knee. If the kneecap is abnormally low, it is a patella baja. Restriction at the back of the knee can prevent it from straightening fully, holding it in fixed flexion deformity.

Pain and complications

Unusual or unexplained swelling, pain and stiffness in the knee can result from inflammation caused by food intolerance (p. 11); inflammatory conditions like rheumatoid arthritis (p. 12); infections from bites or cuts; circulatory problems; diseases (including illnesses like tuberculosis and sexually transmitted diseases, p. 13); hormonal problems (p. 14); or bone disease.

Sometimes knee swelling occurs because gravity brings excess fluid down from higher up the leg, perhaps as a result of injury in the thigh muscles or the hip region. Pain can also be transferred to the knee from other parts of the body: hip problems, especially in children, can cause pain which seems localized to the knee.

Knee injuries

The knee is probably the joint most often injured through sport. Any of the knee's structures can be injured through trauma or overuse at any age. Knee movement and stability can be undermined when the leg bones grow, especially in the teens. They also deteriorate with age, unless you do the right exercises to maintain them.

Knee injuries affect the whole leg, and, through compensation, the hip and knee on the opposite side.

Traumatic bone injury

The weight-bearing bones of the knee can be broken or cracked through trauma at any age. A major fracture can happen together with dislocation of the main knee joint. In young children the femoral or tibial epiphyses (growth areas) can be damaged.

What you feel
There is immediate pain, and there may be obvious displacement of the bones, with swelling, bruising and sometimes bleeding. Shock can set in after the accident. You cannot move the knee or put weight on it.

Causes
A violent force, such as a fall with a heavy load pressing on the leg, causes fracture. The bones break more easily if they are weakened by mineral deficiency or bone conditions such as osteoporosis.

Directions
You must be treated in hospital as an emergency. You may need surgery to realign and stabilize the bones. Otherwise the leg may be immobilized in a plaster cast. You will have to rest in bed for the first phase of healing. You will need to use crutches when you are first allowed on your feet. You may be able to take full weight through your leg within 3–6 months of the accident.

How long?
At least a year.

Cartilage (meniscus) tear

The menisci can be damaged or torn through a sudden force in an acute traumatic injury, or through repetitive attrition in an overuse injury. A cartilage can split across its width or down its length. Cysts can form on a cartilage. There may be damage to one or both cartilages, and sometimes to other tissues as well, including the cruciate or collateral ligaments.

Meniscus damage can happen at any age, but is least common in very young children. Overuse meniscus damage tends to happen from late middle age onwards. In children plica syndrome causes symptoms similar to those of meniscus damage, but the problem is caused by folds of synovial tissue getting damaged or trapped inside the knee.

What you feel
The acute phase is usually very painful. The knee may not swell up immediately, but may become puffy some time after the injury. At a later stage, if the injury becomes chronic, there may be swelling after walking, running or sports. In both the traumatic tear and the overuse injury, if there is pain, it usually occurs on certain movements, especially when the knee is twisted. There may be a sensation of clicking or catching. Sometimes the knee locks, usually in the bent position, so you have to shake it or manipulate it with your hands to free it. The joint may tend to give way if you try to walk or run, especially going down stairs, changing direction, or on uneven ground. The knee might feel hot or unusually cool.

The Knee

Causes

An acute cartilage tear is usually caused by a sudden twisting movement when the knee is under load, as can happen while running and turning, particularly if your foot gets stuck. Cartilage tear can also happen when the knee is straight, for instance if you jump from a height and land heavily on the leg. Children are more vulnerable to meniscus trauma if they have a discoid cartilage, where the centre of the cartilage is thicker than normal.

Overuse cartilage damage can happen through excessive repetitive pressure. It is more likely to happen if the mechanical efficiency of your knee has been undermined by your activities, poor postural habits or previous injury.

Directions

With meniscus damage or plica syndrome, you may need surgery to repair or remove damaged tissue. If possible, it is best to take some time beforehand to regain muscle function and joint mobility. Either you will recover full fitness, or you will be better prepared for an eventual operation.

Surgery is usually done as an arthroscopy, through a 'keyhole', so it does not involve cutting a large scar through the skin. It is often done under epidural anaesthesia, so you remain conscious and avoid the possible side effects of a full anaesthetic. Recovery is deceptively quick after arthroscopy. You may be discharged from hospital the same day. You may be advised that you can return to running and sports within two to three weeks. However, it is never a good idea to rush back to normal activities. The knee may look and feel quite normal, but if you have not done a complete rehabilitation programme, your proprioception mechanisms will not function properly. The knee will also be slightly weak and possibly stiff, causing compensation movements elsewhere in the body. That can lead to problems later, including degenerative arthritis (osteoarthritis).

How long?

6 weeks to 6 months.

Cruciate ligament damage

One or both cruciate ligaments can be torn, partly torn or strained traumatically. Injury can happen in isolation or in conjunction with damage to other tissues. The cruciates can also suffer overuse injury through repetitive stress, especially if the knee has suffered previous injuries. Cruciate ligament injury happens mostly to teenagers and adults up to middle age, and is least common in very young children.

What you feel

If both cruciates tear, there is severe pain and the knee becomes unstable with a 'floppy' feeling. When one cruciate tears there is usually a sharp 'crack', but often surprisingly little pain. If you try to carry on with your sport, you find the knee is unstable.

If a cruciate ligament is partly torn, strained or worn, the knee may feel weak and unstable in specific situations. When you stand still and turn slightly sideways, the knee feels as if it could give way. It can feel painful and swell up during or after sport.

Causes

Traumatic injury usually involves a sudden violent twisting, wrenching or jarring force, while overuse injury results from attritional twisting and jarring. The cruciates are more prone to injury if there is muscle imbalance around the knee, or if dietary deficiency has weakened the ligaments.

Directions

If the injury is severe, surgery may be needed, either immediately or later. There are many different kinds of operation to repair cruciate ligament tears. Most surgeons take tissue from elsewhere in the body to make a graft, while some use synthetic materials. If the surgery is done well, there should be no reason why you should not return to a reasonable level of sporting activity.

Without surgery, it is possible to recover adequate function in a cruciate-deficient knee, if you strengthen the surrounding muscles, especially the hamstrings, sufficiently to compensate for the damaged cruciate.

In all cases protective exercises should be continued indefinitely. Even after a good recovery, you may need a specially designed brace for high-risk sports like skiing.

How long?

4–12 months.

Kneecap pain ('runner's knee')

Pain over the kneecap area on the front of the knee is referred to by various names, including 'runner's knee', kneecap pain syndrome, chondromalacia patellae, anterior knee pain, patellofemoral pain syndrome, retropatellar pain, patellar malalignment syndrome, patellar chondropathy, retropatellar arthritis or arthrosis, patellar arthralgia and patellalgia.

It can come on suddenly as the result of trauma, but is often a gradual overuse injury. It is an extremely common problem which can happen at any age to sporting and non-sporting people alike. Teenage girls are considered especially vulnerable to kneecap pain.

The pain is not specifically related to damage inside the knee or on the back of the kneecap. There may or may not be damage such as arthritic change or roughening of the bone cartilage. In the young there may be softening and pitting in the cartilage surface of the bone, technically called chondromalacia patellae. In older age there may be degenerative arthritis (osteoarthritis). If damage is evident on a scan or X-ray, it does not necessarily cause pain: it can be present without hurting. Conversely, there may be severe symptoms typical of the syndrome, without any visible damage to the joint surfaces to explain it.

What you feel

The pain can be sudden and sharp, like a stabbing or searing sensation when you put your weight on the leg and bend the knee. It can make you stop in your tracks or limp. More often the pain is a dull ache, sometimes like a 'gnawing' sensation in the front of the knee. The knee makes a clicking or grating sound when you bend or straighten it. Any pressure which constricts the kneecap, such as tight jeans or bandaging, causes pain.

Holding the knee bent for long periods is painful. Sitting makes the knee ache – the so-called 'cinema' or 'movie-goer's sign'. There may be a sharp pain as you stand up after sitting still, and also when the knee bends under the load of your body weight, especially going up and down stairs, kneeling or crouching, walking or running on hilly or rough ground, or cycling with the saddle too low. Sometimes the pain comes on after activity or during the night.

Causes

Traumatic injury is often caused by a direct blow to the kneecap. Overuse injury relates to activities which use the knee in a bent position without allowing it to straighten fully, such as running, especially downhill, cycling with the saddle too low, breaststroke swimming, prolonged squatting, or sitting with your knee(s) bent for long periods. Previous injury to another part of the knee can lead to kneecap pain if you have not rehabilitated properly.

Other influences include hip problems, stiff hips, general joint stiffness or hypermobility, faulty foot mechanics, and leg growth, especially in the teenage years.

The key factor in kneecap pain is malfunction in the VMO muscle. It can be weak, wasted and therefore difficult to activate, or sometimes it is in a state of constant tension and cannot be released. In either case the result is poor tracking of the kneecap, which is pulled or held towards the knee's outer side.

Tip: Avoid the squat-sitting exercise, resting against a wall with your hips and knees bent at right angles, which is often recommended for knee strengthening before skiing.

Directions

You must avoid any activities which hold the knee bent or cause pain. In the early stages a small strap just below the kneecap can help discomfort when you walk. You may be fitted with orthotics if foot mechanics are a factor.

In a chronic case you may be offered an operation, usually a lateral release, in which the tissues at the outer side of the knee are cut, to allow better positioning of the kneecap. Some surgeons use more drastic interventions.

In every case you will need to work on restoring and maintaining VMO function.

How long?

A few days to 12 months.

Kneecap traumatic fracture

The patella can be cracked or broken apart in a traumatic injury at any age. The attachment point of the patellar tendon is vulnerable to avulsion fracture, in which violent stress on the tendon pulls the bone apart.

What you feel
There is sudden pain, usually swelling and sometimes bleeding. Bruising appears later on. Movements which stress the kneecap and direct pressure on the bone hurt. You may be able to put weight through your leg, but walking is difficult.

Causes
Fracture can be caused by a wrench when the knee is bent, or a direct blow. Fractures happen more easily if your bones are weakened by mineral deficiency or osteoporosis.

Directions
If the patella is badly separated, you may need an operation to put it together, which usually involves threading a wire through the broken parts. The wire may or may not be removed at a later stage. Without surgery, the knee may be immobilized in a splint or possibly a plaster cast until the bone has healed. You will need crutches at first.

Bone healing time varies according to the individual. Normally, a bone like the patella which does not take body weight directly has a primary healing phase of about ten days. Within three weeks there may be reunion of the fractured parts, and new bone (callus) forming round the crack(s). From six to twelve weeks the bone strengthens. You should avoid stressing the knee, especially bending it under load, until the bone is fully healed.

How long?
6–12 months.

Kneecap dislocation and subluxation

The patella can be pulled out of place: if it pops back quickly, the injury is a subluxation, but if it stays out, it is a dislocation. This traumatic injury can happen at any age, but is particularly common among teenage girls.

What you feel
In a dislocation there is extreme pain and you cannot move the knee. In a subluxation the knee usually hurts, but you may be able take some weight through the leg. In either case the knee is painful to touch, and there may be a lot of swelling, sometimes also bruising, immediately or later on.

Causes

These injuries are usually the result of a violent force when the knee is bent and twisted. Malfunction in the VMO is a key factor, and the injury is often associated with weakness in the calf or thigh muscles, or stiffness in the ankles or hips. In the young, especially teenagers, development of the pelvic bones and leg length growth can play a part.

Directions

A major dislocation should be treated in hospital as an emergency. If the kneecap keeps dislocating or subluxing, you may need an operation to stabilize it. In all cases you have to work on stabilizing the knee, especially by strengthening the VMO. Orthotics may help if your foot movements are faulty. Protective exercises must be maintained indefinitely.

How long?

Several months.

Kneecap stress fracture

Overuse can cause a crack in the patella at any age. In children the condition known as bipartite or tripartite patella is very similar to a stress fracture: repetitive stress disrupts the growth points at the corners of the kneecap so the separate parts fail to fuse when they should, or are pulled apart.

What you feel

The front of the knee aches after any exercise which puts weight through the bent knee, such as crouching, or running, especially on hills, camber or bends. You may find a tender spot or line if you hold the kneecap steady and press gently down it. With rest the pain settles quickly, but it returns with increasing severity if you continue the activities which caused it, until eventually you have to stop. There may be aching at night, but in general the knee is pain-free when you are not exercising. If the patellofemoral joint mechanics are disrupted, you will also have the symptoms of kneecap pain syndrome.

Causes

Any unaccustomed activity which repetitively stresses the bent knee under load can cause a patellar stress fracture. It is a common problem in young army recruits who start training by running long distances day after day in stiff boots on uneven terrain. It happens more easily if the bone is weakened due to mineral deficiency or disease.

Directions

You must rest from pain-causing activities and sports for long enough to allow the bone to heal, which usually takes six to eight weeks. Meanwhile you should do gentle exercises, especially for the VMO, and alternative training to stimulate healing. You may need crutches in the first instance if walking has become painful. You should allow two more weeks after the bone has healed before making a gradual return to sport.

How long?

3–6 months.

Prepatellar bursitis ('housemaid's knee')

Any of the bursae around the knee can become inflamed or suffer damage through trauma or overuse at any age. The bursa which lies under the skin over the kneecap is most often affected. If the skin is broken, the bursa can become infected.

What you feel
Prepatellar bursitis causes an egg-like swelling on the knee which may or may not be painful to touch, but which can cause pain when you bend the knee, especially if you put pressure on it with a tight bandage or by kneeling. If the bursa is very inflamed, it can feel hot and look reddened.

Causes
Trauma is usually a direct blow or kick to the kneecap. Overuse is most often due to repetitive irritation through kneeling or crouching for long periods, so carpet layers, floor tilers and gardeners are at particular risk.

Directions
Your doctor may aspirate the fluid. In a severe case the bursa may be removed surgically, after which your knee has to be protected according to your practitioner's instructions. More often the bursa recovers if you avoid painful movements and direct pressure, use arnica or heparinoid cream around the swelling (p. 29) and do rehabilitation exercises. Sometimes the swollen bursa remains enlarged, but if it is not painful and does not interfere with your knee function, it can be ignored.

How long?
2–4 months.

Medial ligament injury

The ligament on the inner side of the knee can be injured through trauma or overuse at any age. It can be completely or partly torn, or strained to varying degrees. Because the medial ligament is attached to the medial meniscus, the two are often injured together. Sometimes the pes anserinus is also injured. If the ligament is badly strained at its attachment on the femur, little flakes of calcium can form in it, a condition known as Pellegrini-Stieda syndrome. In young children medial ligament injury can accompany a crack in the femoral or tibial epiphyses.

What you feel
In a traumatic injury there is sudden pain on the inner side of the knee, tenderness on pressure, possibly some swelling, and the joint may feel unstable or 'loose'. When the ligament is strained, there is pain, often quite sharp, when the knee is twisted a certain way, even if only slightly. The injured area may feel uncomfortable if you lie on one side with your knees touching.

Causes
There is usually a twisting strain which opens up the inner side of the knee when your weight is on the leg. Overuse strain happens through repetitive twisting, which may be very slight. This is a particular risk of breaststroke swimming, and can happen to racing cyclists if the pedals are not adjusted properly. In runners the problem can be linked to inappropriate shoes or faulty foot mechanics. Imbalance round the hip or ankle can contribute.

Directions

You may need surgery if you have a complete tear or Pellegrini-Stieda syndrome, or if the medial meniscus is involved, while in a more minor injury the knee is usually protected from twisting movements in a splint and rehabilitated. You should correct any contributory factors due to faulty equipment or biomechanical imbalance.

How long?

3–12 months.

Lateral ligament injury

The lateral ligament can be injured traumatically at any age, but is less vulnerable to overuse injuries than the medial ligament or the iliotibial tract. If it is torn or badly damaged, other structures may be injured too. An isolated injury usually involves only minor damage.

What you feel

There is pain on the outer side of the knee when the joint is twisted, and the ligament feels tender if you press it. There may be localized swelling. There is usually little pain at rest.

Causes

A violent twisting movement can overstretch the ligament, especially if the knee is forced outwards.

Directions

The knee is usually protected in soft bandaging or a splint in the acute phase. More rarely, if it is badly torn, it might need surgery.

How long?

3–12 weeks.

Iliotibial tract (band) friction syndrome

Just above the outer side of the knee, the iliotibial tract and its underlying bursa can become irritated through overuse. The injury can happen at any age, but is least common in children.

What you feel

Pain usually comes on gradually during a repetitive activity such as distance running or cycling. Typically, aching starts after a certain time, often about ten minutes, and usually eases off towards the end of the session. There is no pain at rest or during other sports like hockey or squash which involve varied leg movements. If you continue repetitive training, the pain gets worse. Eventually you may even have pain walking. There is tenderness at a certain angle, usually about 30 degrees, if you press over the painful area and bend and straighten your knee gently, and there may also be a snapping sensation.

Causes

Biomechanical inefficiency is a major factor, especially stiffness in the hip, bow-leggedness (genu varum), excessive supination in the foot, or sometimes overpronation. Running on a camber, or a change of running shoes, bicycle or cycling pedals can trigger the problem.

Directions
Rehabilitation exercises focus on stretching the iliotibial tract through the hip abductor muscles and mobilizing the hip (p. 164), as well as strengthening the VMO. Biomechanical factors must be corrected. If your foot mechanics are faulty, orthotics may help. You may be advised to have surgery if the bursa becomes particularly large and inflamed.

How long?
2 weeks to 4 months.

Popliteus strain

The popliteus tendon can be strained through overuse, sometimes causing inflammation in its synovial sheath. The lateral cartilage may also be involved. The injury can happen at any age.

What you feel
The symptoms can be very similar to those of the iliotibial tract friction syndrome, but you may also feel pain when you bend the knee fully, especially if you crouch down. You may find a tender spot if you sit and put your ankle over the opposite knee, and press hard on the outer side or back of the painful knee.

Causes
The causes are often similar to those for iliotibial tract friction syndrome. Popliteus can also be strained if you do a lot of crouching and twisting movements, such as limbo dancing.

Directions
Surgery may be needed if the cartilage is involved.

How long?
3–12 weeks.

Popliteal bursitis – 'Baker's cyst'

Any of the bursae behind the knee can become inflamed and swollen, usually through overuse, at any age. If the skin is broken, the bursa can become infected.

What you feel
The swollen bursa usually causes pressure at the back of the knee, which may or may not be painful, but which makes it difficult to bend and straighten the joint.

Causes
Unfamiliar internal pressure is often a cause, for instance when a runner changes running style, or a rower alters foot position in a rowing boat. The problem can come on in conjunction with other knee injuries, including meniscus damage.

Directions
Your doctor may drain the excess fluid from the bursa. In a severe case the bursa may be surgically excised. Contributory factors must be corrected, and orthotics may help in some cases.

How long?
3–6 months.

Osteoarthritis (osteoarthrosis)

The bone cartilage surfaces inside the knee can be damaged through wear-and-tear arthritis. There may be loss of joint space, causing a visible deformity such as bow leg, knock-knee or fixed flexion deformity. One or both knees may be affected. The problem usually becomes apparent around the age of fifty, but may be evident much earlier, in the thirties, or even the late twenties.

What you feel
There may be pain during or after strenuous or repetitive activities which stress the knee. There is usually pain at night. The knee may swell up and feel stiff after sport or when you sit or stand still for long periods. Movements gradually become more limited, so you find it difficult or impossible to bend or straighten the knee fully. The symptoms are not necessarily related to the degree of damage visible in the joint. A severely arthritic knee can be painless and fully functional.

Causes
Failure to rehabilitate the knee fully after injury is a major cause of later painful osteoarthritis. It is a big risk for professional footballers and other sports players who return to competition too soon after injury: they have a high incidence of early onset osteoarthritis. Degenerative changes are more likely after an injury which has caused bleeding into the joint for a length of time, or if you have a hereditary tendency to osteoarthritis. Sports which put a lot of strain on the knees, such as long-distance running, powerlifting and skiing, can lead to osteoarthritis if you fail to do exercises to maintain full mobility and good muscle balance round the joints, both during your sporting career and later on as you get older.

Directions
Treatments are aimed at controlling the symptoms. You have to avoid painful activities, so you may have to reduce or stop sports involving running, jumping or contact. You also have to avoid being still for long periods. Any painless activities, especially cycling, swimming, tai chi and yoga, can help your knees.

If the symptoms are severe, you may be offered injections or tablets. Remember that pain relief is not the same as functional cure, so if you continue activities like long-distance running you are likely to cause further damage. The last resort is knee replacement surgery.

In all cases it is vital to improve your knee strength, stability and mobility. Protective exercises should be continued indefinitely.

How long?
This is a long-term condition.

Rehabilitation and recovery

Acute phase

You should use the circulatory care measures (p. 27) according to your practitioner's instructions. The basic exercises for the vastus medialis obliquus start as soon as possible, and your practitioner may use electrical muscle stimulation for the VMO as well. Do the VMO exercises on both legs, even if only one knee is injured, because the extra stress on your good leg can disrupt its VMO function.

You may need crutches at first (p. 32). If you use a knee support, it should extend about 15 centimetres (six inches) above and below the knee, or from ankle to thigh if there is a lot of swelling and pain. You can wrap the knee in cotton wool padding, covering it with one or two crepe bandages to provide soft but firm support. Alternatively you can use a ready-made knee support with straps to allow for adjusting the size.

Tip: Avoid using an enclosed tubular support bandage – the kind you pull on like a sleeve – as it can restrict the circulation and weaken the VMO. It should only be used for very short periods, if at all.

Early phase

In all cases the priority is to restore efficient function in the VMO and the muscle groups which coordinate with it. You should add the advanced VMO exercises to the basic ones. For cruciate ligament injuries or hyperextending knees, you should also do the hamstring-emphasis strengthening programme.

As soon as you can, when your practitioner allows, you should do alternative training (p. 25), and start to work on the full front-thigh stretch (p. 126), basic front-thigh strengthening exercises (p. 127) and the knee mobilizing exercises, within pain limits. When you can take weight through your leg, you should start the exercises for correct walking (p. 34), balance (p. 36) and soleus strength (p. 82, exercise 4). Aim at two to three sessions daily.

Recovery phase

Once your knee is stable, when you have regained control of the VMO and can lock the knee straight, you can progress to the straight-leg raising exercises, including the straight-leg raise lying on your side (p. 162, exercise 3). Keep doing all the VMO exercises.

When your knee is pain-free, add weight-resisted, weight-bearing and advanced strengthening exercises for the calf (p. 82), front thigh (p. 128), hamstrings (p. 137), inner thigh (p. 146) and

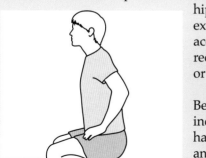

hip (p. 166). You should also do stretching and mobilizing exercises for these areas, but avoid hamstring stretching, according to your practitioner's instructions, if you are recovering from problems involving the cruciate ligaments or hyperextension of the knee.

Before progressing to the final recovery phase (p. 308), including running and sport-related activities, you must have regained efficiency in the VMO, front-thigh flexibility, and front-thigh and hamstring strength, and you should be able to squat fully.

Re-injury prevention

For injury prevention and long-term maintenance, keep up a daily routine of leg exercises, especially those for the VMO and hamstrings.

If you cannot regain the full squat, you should avoid or reduce potentially damaging sporting activities like skiing, football, squash, hard-court tennis, fencing and long-distance running. You should keep yourself fit with cycling, swimming, balanced weight training or any activities which do not cause a reaction of pain, stiffness or swelling in the knee.

Electrical muscle stimulation for the VMO

Knee pain, whatever the cause, results in instant inhibition in the VMO. Getting the VMO to function again is not easy, as the other, bigger parts of the quadriceps group take over and make it difficult for the nerve signals to reach this small muscle. It is very difficult to regain the VMO's nerve-muscle coordination through exercises alone. Electrical muscle stimulation (EMS, p. 20) is invaluable for retraining VMO function, and your practitioner may show you how to use it as a self-help treatment at home. Even after recovery, EMS can be used to maintain precise function in the VMO.

Essential VMO exercises

1. **Patellar twitch**. Sitting on the floor or on the edge of a chair, with your leg straight and foot turned slightly outwards (preferably wearing shorts so that you can see your knees), tighten your thigh muscles very slightly to draw the kneecap upwards on the thigh, keeping the outer-thigh muscles relaxed; then release the knee so that the kneecap glides downwards and is loose – you should be able to move the kneecap from side to side when it is relaxed. 5–10 times on each leg in turn. *Variation: when this is easy, repeat the exercise standing up.*

2. **Knee hyperextension, sitting**. Sitting on the floor or on the edge of a chair, with your leg straight and foot turned slightly outwards, tighten your thigh muscles, straightening your knee as hard as you can; relax completely. 5–10 times on each leg in turn.

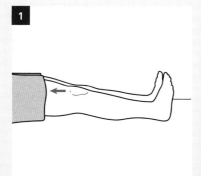

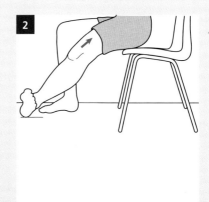

Advanced VMO exercises

1. **Knee hyperextension, standing**. Standing with your legs straight, tighten your thigh muscles to straighten your knee as hard as you can; relax completely. 5–10 times on each leg in turn.

2. **Leg extension, stomach-lying**. Lying on your stomach, lock your knee straight and lift the leg up a little way behind you; check that the knee is still locked by tightening the thigh muscles again, hold for a count of 3, then lower the leg and relax completely. 5–10 times.

3. **Knee hyperextension, stomach-lying**. Lying on your stomach, with your toes tucked so that you balance on the balls of the feet, straighten your knees as hard as you can, then relax completely. 5–10 times.

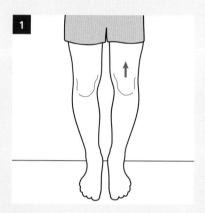

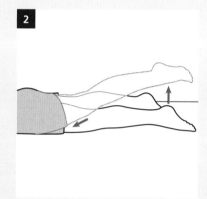

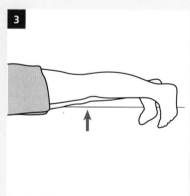

Knee mobilizing exercises

1. **Slide-bending**. Sitting on the floor with your legs resting on a smooth board sprinkled with talcum powder, slide your heel gently towards your bottom and back again. 10–20 times.

2. **High-sitting self-assisted bending**. Sitting on a high chair or bench, support your injured leg with the good leg and gently bend and straighten the good leg rhythmically as far as you comfortably can. 10–20 times.

3. **Prone-lying self-assisted bending**. Lying on your stomach, support your injured leg with your good leg under the ankle, then gently bend and straighten the good leg rhythmically as far as you comfortably can. 10–20 times.

4. **Bicycle bending**. With the saddle high, resistance off, sit on an exercise bicycle and turn the pedals backwards and forwards as far as you comfortably can. You will probably do a full turn backwards before you can do it forwards. Once you can do the full turn forwards, lower the saddle and repeat.

5. **Knee rotation**. Sitting on a chair with your legs about 23 centimetres (nine inches) apart, feet flat on the floor, turn your feet inwards and outwards as far as you can, pivoting on your heels; use your hands to keep your thighs as still as possible, and aim to make the movements symmetrical on both sides. 10–20 times.

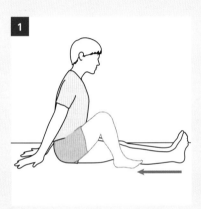

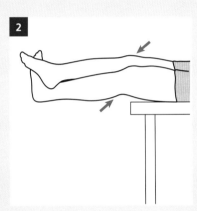

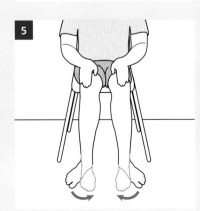

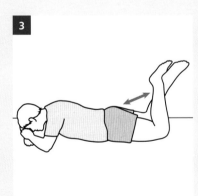

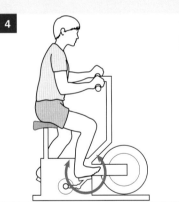

Straight-leg raise exercises

1. **Straight-leg raise**. Sitting on the floor with your legs straight, or lying on your back, lock your knee, keeping your foot turned slightly outwards, lift the leg up as far as you can with the knee locked absolutely straight; hold for a count of 3, then slowly lower the leg and relax completely. 5–10 times.

2. **Straight-leg raise with hip rotation**. Lying on your back, or sitting with your back supported, legs straight and feet turned slightly outwards, tighten the thigh muscles of your leg, straightening the knee as hard as you can; lift the leg upwards and outwards, keeping the foot turned out, knee locked; make 3 circles in the air, then return to the starting position and relax. 5–10 times.

3. **Straight-leg raise with hip adduction and abduction**. Lying on your back, lock your knee straight; keeping it locked, lift your leg straight up, across the other leg, out to the side, back to centre, then slowly lower the leg and relax. 5–10 times.

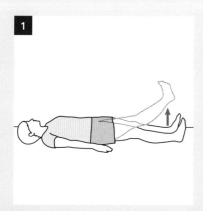

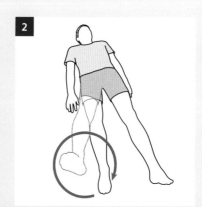

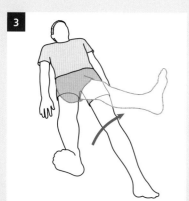

Hamstring-emphasis strengthening programme

1. **Isometric middle range**. Sitting on an upright chair with your hips and knees at right angles, and the heel of your injured leg against the chair leg, press the back of your heel against the chair leg for a count of 5, then relax completely. 3–6 times.

2. **Isometric middle range for the lateral hamstring**. Sitting on an upright chair with your hips and knees at right angles, the heel of your injured leg against the chair leg and your foot turned outwards, press the back of your heel against the chair leg for a count of 5, keeping your foot turned out, then relax completely. 3–6 times.

3. **Isometric inner range**. Sitting forwards towards the edge of an upright chair so that your knee forms an acute angle, with the heel of your injured leg against the chair leg, press the back of your heel against the chair leg for a count of 5, then relax completely. 3–6 times.

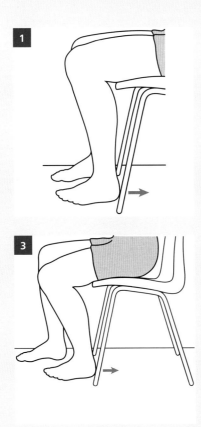

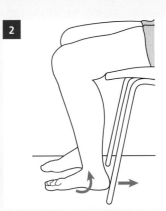

9

The Front-Thigh Muscles

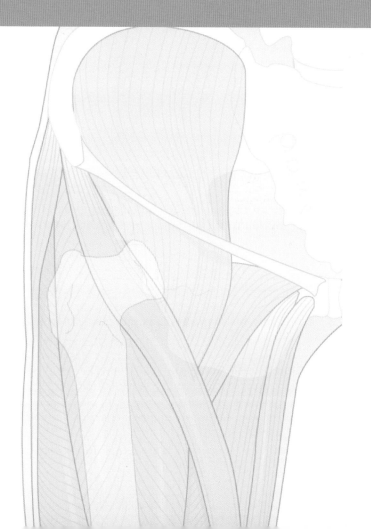

The Front-Thigh Muscles

RIGHT THIGH, FRONT VIEW.

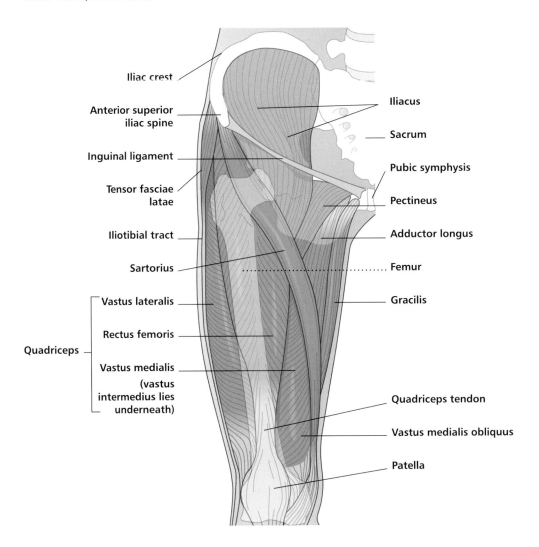

Iliac crest

Anterior superior iliac spine

Inguinal ligament

Tensor fasciae latae

Iliotibial tract

Sartorius

Vastus lateralis

Rectus femoris

Quadriceps

Vastus medialis (vastus intermedius lies underneath)

Iliacus

Sacrum

Pubic symphysis

Pectineus

Adductor longus

Femur

Gracilis

Quadriceps tendon

Vastus medialis obliquus

Patella

The front thigh consists of the quadriceps muscle group and the sartorius muscle, which lie over and around the femur (thigh bone), and a small muscle called articularis genus (p. 98).

Structure

The femur is a major weight-bearing bone containing bone marrow. It forms part of the hip at its upper end, and the knee at its lower end.

Quadriceps means 'four-headed': there is no such thing as a 'quadricep'. The four parts forming this muscle group are vastus lateralis on the outer side of the thigh, vastus intermedius, the deepest-lying muscle covering the central area, vastus medialis along the inner side of the front thigh, and rectus femoris, the most superficial part, which forms a line from the front of the ilium (hip bone) down to the knee.

The four quadriceps muscles come together into the quadriceps tendon above the kneecap and cover the bone (p. 97). The vastus medialis forms horizontal fibres called the vastus medialis obliquus (VMO, p. 99) at its lower end, which bind to the inner side of the patella, whereas the other parts of quadriceps form strong attachments over the top and outer side of the bone. From the lower tip of the patella, the quadriceps tendon forms the patellar tendon (ligamentum patellae), a short tough band which is attached to the tibial tubercle on the front of the tibia. When your leg is straight and relaxed, you can move the kneecap around with your hand. You can feel the patellar tendon best when the knee is bent.

Sartorius is the longest muscle in the body. Its upper end is attached to the front of the ilium above the rectus femoris, and passes downwards towards the inner side of the knee. Its lower end is fixed to the top of the front inner edge of the tibia, where its tendon forms part of the pes anserinus (p. 98).

What they do

The quadriceps muscles are active when you walk, run, jump or kick.

Acting concentrically against gravity or a load, quadriceps shortens to straighten the knee, for instance when you stand up from crouching or sitting, go up steps, push down on bicycle pedals or pull through to back stops in a rowing boat. Working eccentrically in the direction of gravity, it pays out to control the opposite movements so that you do not collapse under the pressure of gravity, for example when you squat down.

Because it encloses the kneecap, quadriceps acts to draw the bone upwards whenever the knee is straightened, and pays out to release it as the knee bends. The horizontal fibres of the VMO play a vital part in controlling the kneecap from the inner side.

Sartorius bends the hip and knee into flexion against gravity, as well as taking the leg out sideways from the hip and rotating it outwards (laterally). These movements are used in classical ballet, meditation sitting in the lotus position, kicking a football with the inner side of the foot, sprinting, walking up stairs and getting on to a car seat.

Rectus femoris also flexes the hip, bending the thigh on the pelvis. It is active together with sartorius and the hip flexors as you take the thigh forwards in walking or running.

Pain and complications

Causes of unexplained pain in the front thigh include circulatory problems, symptoms referred from the back or hip, or, rarely, a tumour.

Front-thigh injuries

The bone, muscles and tendons in the front thigh can be torn, partly torn or strained through trauma or overuse at any age. In any knee injury, the muscles are weakened dramatically. The VMO is inhibited immediately, while the rest of the front-thigh muscles weaken and shrink during the first few hours.

Front-thigh injuries have a direct effect on the hip and knee, and can cause disruption to the rest of the leg, the lower back and the other leg.

Femoral traumatic fracture

The thigh bone can be broken or cracked through trauma. The bone ends can stay close together in a stable fracture, or separate to become unstable. Fracture can happen at any age. In young children fractures of the shaft are often greenstick, in which one side of the bone breaks, while the other side is distorted but does not give way, or they can affect the epiphyses (growth areas) at either end of the bone.

What you feel
There is usually a lot of pain, but in some cases surprisingly little. There may be a lot of bleeding, bruising and swelling. You cannot move the leg normally, or take any weight through it. You may lose feeling below the break. Clinical shock can set in.

During recovery you may feel a deep ache in the bone, and you may notice a lumpy swelling over the fracture site, both of which are normal.

Causes
It takes a violent force to break the femur, such as a bad fall with a weight across the leg. Fracture happens more easily if the bone is weakened by mineral deficiency or disease.

Directions
A traumatic fracture has to be treated as an emergency. You may need an operation to realign or stabilize the broken bone, or the leg may be immobilized in a cast. You will probably have to rest in bed for the first phase of recovery. When you are allowed up, you will need to use crutches. The bone gradually heals over three to six months. Weight-bearing must be progressive to minimize the risk of re-fracture.

How long?
15–24 months.

Femoral stress fracture

The thigh bone can crack in any part of its length through overuse stress. The injury can happen at any age, but is least common in children.

What you feel
You may feel an ache after exercise or at night. Pain in the thigh gradually increases if you continue doing the same type of exercise.

Causes
Repetitive muscle pull against the bone causes micro-damage and cracks. The injury is associated with activities like long-distance running, doing drills for high jumping, or overtraining for squat exercises in powerlifting. The risk is increased if you train on consecutive days without doing alternative training or allowing for rest days. A change of routine is usually the trigger, whether an increase in mileage or resuming training after a lay-off. The injury is more likely to happen if your bones are weakened by osteoporosis, disease or mineral deficiency.

Directions
The stress fracture is diagnosed on the basis of your description of your pain and, if necessary, a bone scan. An X-ray does not necessarily reveal a stress fracture in the early stages before it has healed. Rest from pain-causing activities is essential, combined with alternative painless exercise to stimulate the healing processes. The bone must heal before you can resume running or repetitive training, and this usually takes at least three months. You should allow two more weeks after the bone has mended before resuming any stressful weight-bearing activities. Your return to sport has to be very gradual to avoid the risk of a complete fracture.

How long?
6–12 months.

Front-thigh muscle traumatic injury

The muscles can suffer a tear, partial tear or strain of the muscles, deep bruising (contusion) or internal bleeding (haematoma) through trauma. If the injury happens close to an attachment point, especially where rectus femoris and sartorius are attached to the front of the ilium, the bony edge may be pulled away in an avulsion fracture. Injury can happen at any age.

What you feel
There may be a lot of pain or surprisingly little. The area is tender to touch, and there may be swelling. The thigh usually stiffens up later on, and you then experience pain if you try to bend and straighten your knee and hip. Your leg may become numb: this is called a 'dead leg'. If there is severe cramping or muscle spasm, the injury is termed a 'charley horse' or 'corked thigh'. In a complete tear, which is most likely to occur in the rectus femoris muscle, the torn ends may form distinct lumps under the skin with a gap between.

Causes

Violent contact is a common cause, such as being kicked or hit. The front-thigh muscles can also be injured through a blocked movement when you try to straighten your knee against excessive pressure, as in a violent football tackle, or if your foot gets stuck when you are trying to run or jump. Sometimes the trauma is cumulative, for instance when female gymnasts slap their thighs repeatedly against the lower of the asymmetrical bars.

Directions

Surgery may be needed for a severe tear, but more often the leg is protected with bandaging or a cast and rehabilitated. You may need crutches in the first phase of healing.

How long?

3 weeks to 6 months.

Myositis ossificans

Internal bleeding from a traumatic injury can cause deep bruising and a haematoma. In some cases, especially if the periosteum (bone covering) has been damaged, this leads to the formation of bone (calcification) in the muscles, technically called myositis ossificans, or heterotopic bone formation. It can happen at any age, but is rare in young children.

What you feel

A painful hard lump develops in the muscles, usually a few weeks after the initial injury. It gradually gets harder and more painful, and may cause visible swelling. Movements of the thigh are painful, especially when you bend your knee and stretch the front-thigh muscles.

Causes

The exact reason why myositis ossificans occurs in some patients is not certain, but there are known risk factors. Among them are failure to control the initial symptoms of a traumatic front-thigh injury, re-injury, and aggravation of the injury through continuing sports and painful activities. Treatments which inflame the area, especially deep massage, can contribute.

Directions

All painful activities must be avoided. The extra bone normally reduces naturally, although it may not disappear completely. Very gentle progressive exercises to restore flexibility and strength to the muscles are introduced gradually. Surgical removal of the extra bone may be considered after several months if there is still a lot of pain and limitation, but generally it is avoided, as the bone can grow back after an operation.

How long?

Several months, if not long term.

Front-thigh muscle overuse strain

The front-thigh muscles can be partly torn, strained or pulled through overuse at any age. The injury is least common in young children.

What you feel
You feel an ache or pain over the front of the thigh during any activity involving the front-thigh muscles. The injured area feels tender to touch, and hurts when you stretch or contract the muscles. There may be swelling.

Causes
Causes include overtraining or unaccustomed training for sports like long-distance running or cycling, or overdoing exercises like squat jumps, hopping and bounding. The injury can be associated with referred pain from the back or hip, or faulty foot mechanics. Sometimes there is an underlying stress fracture.

Directions
You have to rest from painful activities and do progressive rehabilitation exercises. You may need tests for underlying problems. Contributory factors must be treated and corrected. Orthotics may help if faulty foot mechanics have contributed.

How long?
3 weeks to 3 months.

Patellar tendon tear

The patellar tendon can be torn completely or partly as a sudden traumatic injury. This can happen at any age, but is rare in children. Sometimes the tendon holds firm, but pulls away its attachment point at the tip of the kneecap (p. 105) or the tibial tubercle in an avulsion fracture (p. 92).

What you feel
When the tendon tears completely, the kneecap jumps upwards on the thigh. A partial tear can make the knee feel loose and difficult to control. The tendon feels painful when you try to move the knee in either direction, and is tender to touch.

Causes
A blocked movement when your knee is fully bent can cause overload on the tendon, as in catching your foot on the run-up to a jump, or a blocked tackle in football. Weightlifters and powerlifters can tear the patellar tendon(s) by overloading the weights on squat-lifts. The patellar tendon is more vulnerable to sudden tear if you have been taking bodybuilding drugs, particularly anabolic steroids, or if it has been treated previously with injections.

Directions
A complete tear may need to be repaired surgically, whereas a more minor tear is usually protected in a cast and rehabilitated.

How long?
6–12 months.

The Front-Thigh Muscles

Patellar tendon strain

Overuse injury to the patellar tendon can cause strain in the tendon fibres, which is usually called patellar tendinitis. This can happen at any age. In young patients, usually teenagers, if there is damage at the lower attachment point on the tibial tubercle, it is known as Osgood-Schlatter's condition (p. 92). Attritional damage due to traction at the upper attachment on the patella is called Sinding-Larsen-Johansson syndrome.

What you feel
There is gradually increasing pain, linked to activities which activate or stretch the tendon. There is tenderness on pressure, and you may notice puffiness around the tendon.

Causes
The main cause is overdoing activities which stress the patellar tendon through repeated movements with the knee bent and loaded. Injury is more likely to happen if you are overtired, or when the tendon has been weakened by dietary deficiency, use of certain anabolic drugs, or previous injury to the knee or front thigh.

Directions
You need to avoid painful activities. A patellar strap can help to take pressure off the tendon. You may be offered an injection into the tendon: if so, make sure your practitioner is expert in this, because, if not, there is a strong risk of the tendon rupturing completely some weeks later.

How long?
6 weeks to several months.

Rehabilitation and recovery

Acute phase
Use the circulatory care measures (p. 27), according to your practitioner's instructions. You should start alternative training for the unaffected areas as soon as possible (p. 25).

Early phase
Rehabilitation may start with isometric exercises for the thigh muscles, especially the essential VMO exercises (p. 112), combined with gentle stretching within pain limits. When you can take weight through your leg, you should do the exercises for correct walking (p. 34) and balance (p. 36). Progress to the basic front-thigh stretching and strengthening exercises, alongside basic exercises for the calf (p. 80), hamstrings (pp. 135–136), inner thigh (pp. 144–145), hip (pp. 160–162) and pelvis (pp. 180–181). Add gradually increasing weights or resistance to the strengthening exercises when possible. Aim at two or three sessions daily.

Recovery phase
When you can do the stretching and basic strengthening exercises fully without pain, you should progress to the advanced strengthening exercises for the front thigh and all the related muscle groups. Always stretch the front thigh before and after any other exercises, preferably in the morning and evening as well.

You must regain full strength, flexibility and coordination in the muscles before moving on to the final recovery phase (p. 308).

Front-thigh stretching exercises

Note: If the front-thigh muscles become tight, whether through injury to the front thigh or knee, overexercising, or sitting for long periods, the two-joint muscles sartorius and rectus femoris tighten most of all. That is why it is essential to stretch the front of the hip as well as the knee to keep the front thigh fully pliable.

1. **Full front-thigh stretch**. Lying on your stomach, bend your knee as far as you can and pull your heel towards your bottom, either with your hand round your ankle, or, if you cannot reach, using a strap round your ankle and pulling on the ends of the strap; otherwise you can use your other leg to push with; hold for a count of 6, then relax completely. 5–10 times.

2. **Standing quadriceps and front-knee stretch**. Standing, bend your knee behind you; with your hand round your ankle, pull your heel gently towards your bottom; hold for a count of 6, then relax completely. 5–10 times.

3. **Kneeling stretch**. Kneeling on a soft surface, sit back on your heels and put your hands down next to your feet; lift your hips up and forwards as far as you can, so that you balance on your shins and hands; hold for a count of 6, then relax completely. 5–10 times.

4. **Quadriceps and medial-knee stretch**. Kneeling with your feet placed outwards to the sides of your buttocks, sit back bending your knees as far as is comfortable; hold for a count of 6, then relax completely. 5–10 times.

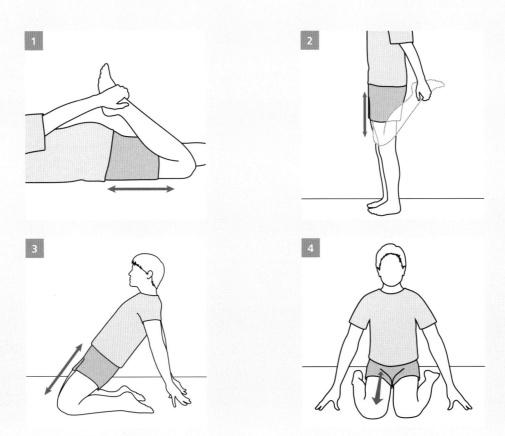

Basic front-thigh strengthening exercises

1. **Knee extension, inner range**. Sitting on a mat on the floor, with a support (e.g. a rolled towel) under your knee, straighten your knee hard to lock it fully, then reverse the movement with control. 5–10 times.

2. **Knee extension**. Using a knee extension machine, or sitting on a support with a rolled towel under your knee, with hips and knees at right angles, straighten the knee to lock it fully, then slowly bend it again. 5–10 times.

3. **Leg extension**. Using a leg press machine, straighten your knees to lock them, then reverse the movement with control. 5–10 times.

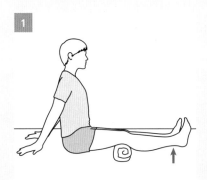

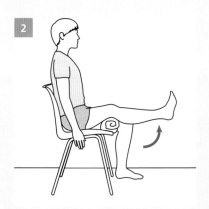

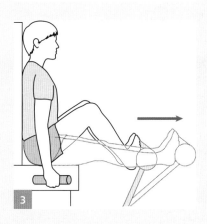

Advanced front-thigh strengthening exercises

Tip: Always lock the knee straight at the end of the movement when you do front-thigh strengthening exercises, to avoid kneecap pain (p. 103).

1. **Stand-ups**. Sitting on a chair, with feet flat and parallel, arms folded, stand up quickly straightening your knees, bend your knees to touch your bottom lightly to the chair, and straighten up again, 5–20 times without stopping.

2. **Mini-squat**. Stand with your back to a low chair or bench, feet slightly apart and parallel, bend your knees with control to touch your bottom to the chair without sitting down; straighten up again quickly and lock your knees once you are upright, then relax the muscles completely. Repeat 5–20 times.

3. **Half-squat**. Standing with your feet slightly apart and parallel, go up on your toes with your knees straight; bend your knees with control to squat halfway down, still on your toes straighten up again quickly and lock your knees, then relax the muscles completely. 5–20 times.

4. **Step-ups**. Standing facing a double step or firm bench, 38–51 centimetres (15–20 inches) high, step up to stand on the bench on both feet, straightening your knees fully, then step down. 10–20 times leading with one foot, then repeat leading with the other foot.

5. **One-legged half-squat**. Standing close to a support on one leg, foot flat, go up on your toes, keeping your knee straight; bend your knee with control to squat halfway down; straighten up again quickly and lock your knee, then relax the muscles completely. 5–10 times.

6. **Full squat**. Standing by a support, go up on your toes; squat down fully with control, keeping your heels up; straighten your knees quickly to stand up, then lower your heels. 5–20 times.

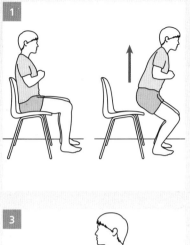

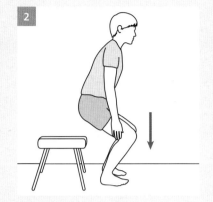

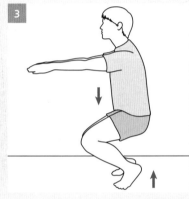

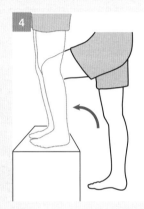

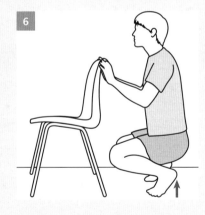

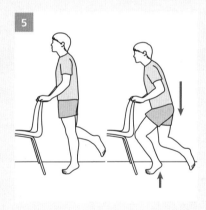

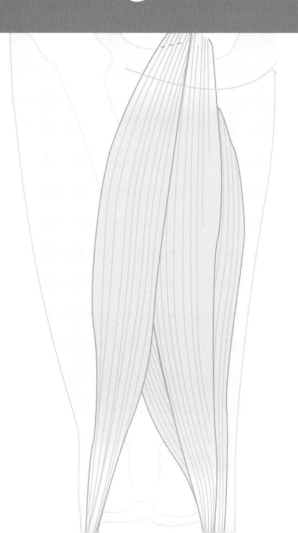

10

The Hamstrings

LEFT THIGH, BACK VIEW.

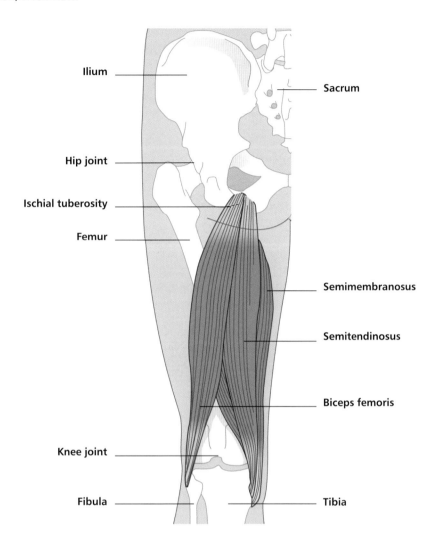

Ilium

Sacrum

Hip joint

Ischial tuberosity

Femur

Semimembranosus

Semitendinosus

Biceps femoris

Knee joint

Fibula

Tibia

The hamstrings are three muscles which cover the back of your thigh, extending from your ischial tuberosity (seat bone) down to the back of your knee. They link the hip and knee joints.

Structure

Semitendinosus has the longest tendon, which is attached at its lower end to the inner side of the top of the tibia at the back of the knee. Underlying semitendinosus is semimembranosus, a fleshier muscle, which is also attached to the inner side of the tibia. These are the medial hamstrings. The third, lateral hamstring, is called biceps femoris, because it has two heads at its upper end. One head forms a common tendon with semitendinosus on the ischial tuberosity, while the other is attached to the back of the femur. Biceps femoris spreads downwards and outwards to attach to the top of the fibula and the top of the tibia at the back of the knee.

The sciatic nerve, which runs centrally down the back of the thigh, supplies all three hamstrings.

Sitting down with your hand on the back of your knee, you can feel the hamstrings contracting as you bend your knee.

What they do

Working concentrically, the hamstrings bend the knee against gravity, and they control the opposite movement, working eccentrically or paying out, when the knee is straightened in the direction of gravity. If you lie on your stomach and bend one knee, the hamstrings perform the movement up to the point where your lower leg is at a right angle to your thigh, and then control the movement if you straighten the knee again. To bend the knee beyond the right angle, the front-thigh muscles control the movement eccentrically against the influence of gravity.

If you are standing up and you keep your thigh absolutely vertical (not an easy thing to do), the hamstrings perform the whole movement of bending your knee and bringing your foot up behind you against gravity, and they control the reverse movement under the influence of gravity.

As they are attached above the hip joint, the hamstrings also extend the hip against gravity when you are standing up or lying on your stomach, and control the reverse movement. This means the hamstrings help the gluteal muscles to take the leg backwards from the hip, and they also help you straighten your trunk from bending forwards while standing up.

When your knee is bent, the medial hamstrings help rotate the knee to turn the foot inwards, while the lateral hamstring turns the foot outwards (p. 99).

The hamstrings are active in walking, running, sprinting, jumping and kicking. They are often relatively weak compared to the front-thigh muscles, which can be a factor in knee injuries. Racing cyclists tend to have more equal hamstring and front-thigh strength than runners or other sports players. Because of their long tendons, the hamstrings tend to tighten easily, whether through overwork as in long-distance running or shortening because of sitting still for long periods.

Cramp in the hamstrings can be a sign of relative dehydration: lying on your stomach, bend one knee fairly quickly about five times. If you get instant cramp in the back of the thigh, you need to drink more water, or, less commonly, take in more salt.

Pain and complications

Sciatica, or 'trapped nerve' (p. 219), is a relatively common cause of pain at the back of the thigh. It can feel like a hamstring strain, and sometimes happens together with a hamstring injury. Unexplained or unusual pain at the back of the thigh can also be due to circulatory problems (p. 12), stress fracture (p. 121), or, very rarely, bone disease, including tumours.

Hamstring injuries

The hamstrings can be torn, partly torn or strained through trauma or overuse at any age. Injury has a direct effect on the calf, knee, hip and lower back.

Traumatic hamstring injury

The hamstring muscles or their tendons can be torn or partly torn in any part of their length. If the damage is close to the attachment on the ischial tuberosity, the bone itself may be pulled away in an avulsion fracture.

What you feel
Injury can result from a sudden overstretch or overcontraction. You may feel or even hear a snap, or you may feel as if you have been kicked in the back of the leg. There may be swelling and bruising, and sometimes a visible gap if the muscle or tendon has torn completely. Walking is painful. In a more minor injury you might feel an unpleasant pulling sensation or irritation. In all cases the area is tender if you press on it, and hurts when you bend or straighten your knee and hip.

Causes
Hamstring tear is relatively common in sprinters, especially if the hamstrings are tight or weak. It can happen through a mistimed kick in football, or through overbalancing or catching your foot in the run-up to a jump. The hamstrings can be overstretched if your foot slides forwards when your leg is straight, for instance if your lead leg slips as you land after jumping a hurdle. These injuries are more likely to happen if you are overtired or dehydrated, or have had a previous injury in the calf, knee, hip or back.

Directions
You may need to use crutches at first. A bad tear might need surgical repair, but more often you simply have to avoid painful activities and follow a rehabilitation programme.

How long?
3–12 weeks.

The Hamstrings

Overuse hamstring injury

A strain or pull in any part of the hamstring muscles or tendons can happen through overuse.

What you feel
There is gradually increasing pain related to sport or training. It may feel like cramp, and may even wear off at times during training, only to return by the end of the session or immediately afterwards. There may be localized tenderness on pressure. At rest there is little or no pain, and walking is usually reasonably comfortable.

Causes
Overtraining in a repetitive sport like distance running, rowing or cycling is often the cause, especially if your hamstrings are weak or tight, or if you have had recent leg injuries. Any change which alters the normal pattern of movement between your foot and thigh can be a trigger, such as altering the footplate in a rowing boat, or running in new shoes on hills or a camber. Dehydration and overtiredness are often factors.

Directions
You must correct any contributory factors. If you do not rehabilitate fully, the problem is likely to recur.

How long?
10 days to several months.

Rehabilitation and recovery

Acute phase
Look after your circulation (p. 27), following your practitioner's advice. If possible, you should do the essential vastus medialis obliquus exercises (p. 112). Alternative training for the unaffected parts of your body should start as soon as possible (p. 25).

Early phase
If you have been using crutches, you should do the exercises for correct walking (p. 34). You need to start stretching the hamstrings very gently, and do the basic strengthening exercises, within pain limits. Isometric hamstring contractions (p. 116) may help specific strength in different parts of the range of movement. You may need to work in outer range at first, pressing the foot down with the knee almost straight, before progressing to middle and inner range. Aim at two or three sessions daily.

Recovery phase
You move on to the advanced hamstring strengthening exercises, together with the advanced VMO exercises (p. 113). You should also do calf (pp. 80–81) and front-thigh (pp. 126–127) stretching and strengthening exercises, exercises for balance (p. 36), basic hip strengthening exercises (p. 162), and strengthening and mobilizing for your pelvis (pp. 180–181). Add gradually increasing weights or resistance for the strengthening exercises when possible. Hamstring stretching should be done before and after any other exercises, preferably morning and evening as well. You need to regain full flexibility, strength and coordination in the muscles before progressing to the final recovery phase (p. 308).

Hamstring stretching exercises

1. **Standing stretch**. Place your heel on a low support; keeping your back straight and head up, lean forwards a little way, with your foot pointing up; when you feel a gentle stretching sensation on the back of the thigh, hold the position for a count of 6, then relax completely. 5–10 times.

2. **Sitting stretch**. Sitting on the floor with one leg straight, and the other bent so that the foot is in contact with the inner thigh of the straight leg, bend forwards from the hips, reaching gently towards your toes, keeping your back straight and head up; hold for a count of 6, then relax completely. 5–10 times.

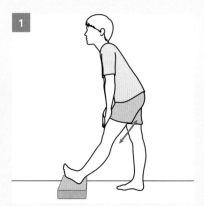

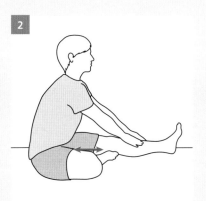

Basic hamstring strengthening exercises

1. **Knee flexion / hamstring curl**. Lying on your stomach on a mat, bend your knee as far as you can, then slowly reverse the movement and relax completely. 5–10 times. Progress to using a weights machine.

2. **Leg extension, stomach-lying**. Lying on your stomach, lock your knee straight and lift the leg up a little way behind you; check that the knee is still locked by tightening the thigh muscles again, hold for a count of 2, then lower the leg and relax completely. 5–10 times.

3. **Standing hip extension**. Standing up straight, move your leg backwards a little way, keeping your back straight and hip well forward; hold for a count of 2, bring the leg forwards to neutral, then take it backwards again without putting your foot down. 10–20 times.

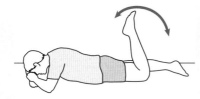

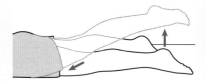

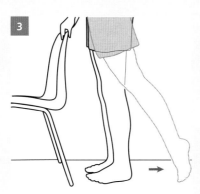

Advanced hamstring strengthening exercises

1. **Standing knee flexion**. Standing up straight, close to a support, bend your knee up behind you quickly, trying to kick your bottom, then reverse the movement more slowly. 10–20 times.

2. **Stomach-lying hip extension with knee bent**. Lying on your stomach with your knee bent to a right angle, lift your leg up backwards from the hip a little way, reverse the movement without putting the leg down completely and repeat. 5–20 times continuously.

3. **Dynamic kick-backs**. Run forwards kicking your heels towards your bottom. 10–50 steps.

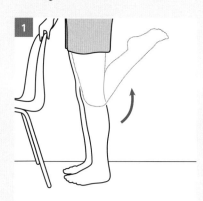

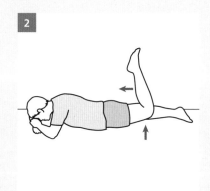

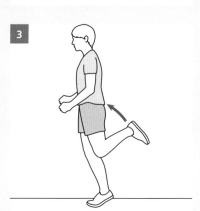

11

The Inner-Thigh Muscles

RIGHT THIGH, FRONT VIEW.

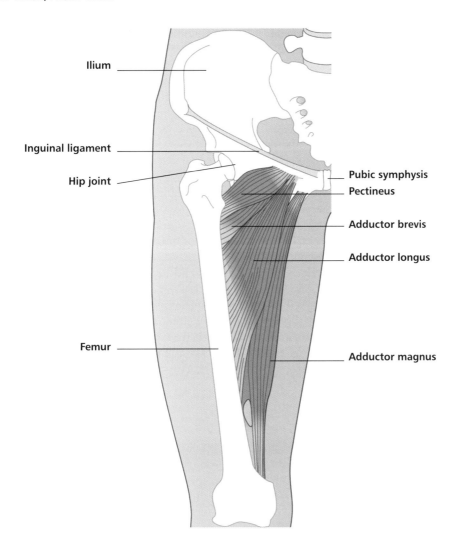

Ilium

Inguinal ligament

Hip joint

Pubic symphysis

Pectineus

Adductor brevis

Adductor longus

Femur

Adductor magnus

The inner or medial thigh comprises five muscles: the three adductors, pectineus and gracilis.

Structure

The adductors are fixed to the lower edge of the pubic bone at the front of the pelvis, and spread out downwards to their attachments along the inner side of the femur.

Adductor longus has a strong cord-like tendon which you can feel and see in the groin area at the top of the inner thigh. It forms the inner edge of a flattened area called the femoral triangle, which you can feel with your hand. The inguinal ligament (p. 169) forms its upper edge, sartorius (p. 119) its outer side, and iliacus and psoas major (p. 149) its deeper part, or floor. The femoral blood vessels and main nerves pass down from the abdominal region to the thigh through the triangle.

Adductor brevis, the smallest of the three adductors, lies behind pectineus and adductor longus and is attached to the edge of the pubic bone and the upper inner side of the femur, behind pectineus. Adductor magnus is a big muscle which lies closest to the midline of the body, behind the other adductors, attaching to the inner part of the pubic bone and the lower inner edge of the femur, just above the condyle, or knuckle. If you put your hand over the lower inner thigh and draw your leg inwards, you can feel the adductor magnus tendon working.

Pectineus is a shorter muscle, lying within the femoral triangle, which links the pecten pubis on the lower front part of the pubic bone to the upper inner edge of the femur. Gracilis lies closer to the surface than the other muscles, and extends from the inner part of the pubic bone, down the inner side of the thigh to the inner edge of the tibia, where it forms part of the pes anserinus (p. 98).

What they do

The adductors draw the thigh inwards against gravity or a resistance, so they are active when you run sideways, kick a ball with the inner side of your foot, or ride a horse. Adductor longus and adductor magnus turn the leg inwards into medial rotation at the hip. Adductor longus is active when the hip flexors bend the leg up at the hip, while adductor magnus contracts during hip extension. Pectineus helps to draw the leg inwards into adduction, and acts to bring the leg forwards into flexion at the hip. Gracilis acts on both the hip and the knee, helping in flexion, adduction and medial rotation.

The adductor muscles compensate if the front-thigh muscles are weak: the legs tend to turn inwards at the hips, for instance if you try to lift excessively heavy weights on a knee extension machine, or if you are running too much. A child who runs with in-turned hips and heels kicking outwards probably has weak thigh muscles and is overtraining. In older age, arthritic changes in the hips and knees are often associated with in-turned hips due to adductor compensation, coupled with muscle weakness and tightness at the front and back of the thigh.

Pain and complications

Unusual or unexplained pain in the groin region can be caused by a hernia (p. 174), a stress fracture in the pubic bones (p. 173), disease affecting the pubic bones, referred symptoms from the back or hip, or an infection or condition which makes the lymph glands in the groin swell and become tender. Pain felt along the inner side of the thigh can be referred from the hip or back. Other causes include bone or muscle disease, circulatory problems or a stress fracture in the femur. Pain from these causes makes the inner-thigh muscles tighten up in spasm, which can seem just like a muscle strain.

Inner-thigh injuries

Any part of the muscles or tendons of the inner-thigh muscles can be injured traumatically or through overuse, at any age. Injury is more likely to happen if your hip is stiff or your knee movement limited. Inner-thigh injury has a direct effect on hip and knee function, impairs function down to the foot, and can cause the other leg to overcompensate.

Inner-thigh traumatic injury

The muscles can be torn, partly torn or strained in any part of their length. If the injury happens close to an attachment point on a bone, the bone may be pulled away in an avulsion fracture.

What you feel
There is usually pain in the injured area, which you feel when you activate or stretch the inner-thigh muscles, as in kicking or running sideways. If there is a tear, there may be bunching of the muscle(s), bruising and localized swelling. The injury feels tender if you press on it. In a strain the symptoms are similar, but there is usually no visible swelling or bruising. The injured muscle(s) may tighten on certain movements, including walking. Most hip movements cause pain, and sometimes certain knee movements also.

Causes
A sudden severe stress which forces your leg out sideways can happen in any sport involving tackling and kicking, high-impact sports like gymnastics, and high-speed sports like downhill skiing or waterskiing. The muscles can overcontract through a blocked movement, or overstretch through overenthusiastic or forced sideways splits. They can be overworked if you run hard up a hill or sprint up stairs.

Directions
You can use ice or cold compresses in the acute phase (p. 29). You need to avoid painful movements, and you should not sit still for long periods. Treatment is usually rehabilitation, but if there is a bad tear you may be offered surgery to mend it.

How long?
3–6 months.

The Inner-Thigh Muscles

Inner-thigh muscle overuse injury

Partial tears and strains can happen in the inner-thigh muscles and their tendons through overuse.

What you feel
There is gradually increasing pain along the inner thigh or in the groin when you do activities which work the muscles and tendons. There is usually some degree of tenderness, and a feeling of tightness in the strained area. Strain of the adductor tendon in the groin can cause a sharp focus of pain and tenderness.

Causes
Excessive training for sports involving kicking or running up slopes can cause strains. Most often the injury is caused by doing unaccustomed training or changing technique in some way. Risk factors include long-distance running on hilly ground, altering your running mechanics with new shoes or orthotics, a new saddle or different horse in horse riding and overtraining in sports involving a sideways run-up, such as cricket bowling, baseball pitching and javelin throwing. Injury happens more easily if you have had previous hip, knee or lower back problems.

Directions
You must correct any contributory factors. For an adductor tendon injury in the groin, you may be offered a pain-relieving injection.

How long?
Muscle strains: 2 weeks to 3 months.
Tendon injury: 1–6 months.

Rehabilitation and recovery

Acute phase
Use the circulatory care measures (p. 27) according to your practitioner's instructions. Alternative training for the unaffected parts of your body should start as soon as possible (p. 25).

Early phase
Once the acute healing phase has passed, you should start doing exercises for correct walking (p. 34). You need to stretch the injured area gently, and do strengthening exercises within pain limits, according to your practitioner's advice. You should combine the exercises with the essential VMO exercises (p. 112), basic strengthening and stretching exercises for the calf (pp. 80–81), front thigh (pp. 126–127) and hip (pp. 160–163), plus strengthening and mobilizing for the pelvis (pp. 180–181). Aim at two to three sessions a day.

Recovery phase
As you recover full flexibility in the injured muscle, you should progress to the advanced inner-thigh strengthening exercises, as well as stretching and strengthening exercises for the calf (p. 82), front thigh (p. 128), hamstrings (p. 137) and hip (pp. 164–166), as well as straight-leg raise (p. 115) and balance (p. 36) exercises. Add gradually increasing weights or resistance for the strengthening exercises when possible. Always stretch the inner-thigh muscles before and after other exercises, and, if possible in the morning and evening.

You must regain full flexibility, strength and coordination in the inner-thigh muscles before progressing to the final recovery phase (p. 308).

Inner-thigh stretching exercises

1. **Sitting stretch with knees straight**. Sitting on the floor with your legs stretched out comfortably sideways and feet turned out, lean forwards from the hips, keeping your back straight and head up, until you feel a slight, gentle stretching sensation along the inner thighs; hold for a count of 6, then relax completely. 3–10 times.

2. **Sitting stretch with knees bent**. Sitting on the floor, place the soles of your feet together, let your knees splay outwards, put your hands round your feet, and rest your elbows against your inner thighs; bring your feet closer to your body using your hands, and press gently against your thighs with your elbows; hold for a count of 6, then relax completely. 3–10 times.

3. **Standing stretch**. Standing with your legs apart, shift your weight sideways, and bend your trunk sideways over the other leg, sliding your hand down the outer thigh, so that you feel a gentle stretch down the inner thigh; hold for a count of 6, then relax completely. 3–10 times.

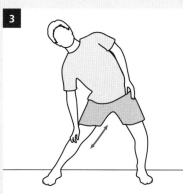

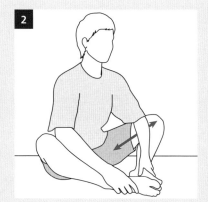

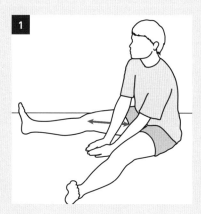

Basic inner-thigh strengthening exercises

1. **Non-weight-bearing isometric strengthener**. Sitting or lying on the floor with your legs straight, place a ball or solid object between your feet, and press your legs together; hold for a count of 5, then relax completely. 3–6 times. Use balls of different sizes to change the range of the exercise.

2. **Isometric strengthener, standing**. Standing sideways, place the inner edge of your foot on a step; press your foot downwards against the step, keeping both legs straight; hold for a count of 5, then relax completely. 3–6 times. To change the range of the contraction, use a higher or lower step.

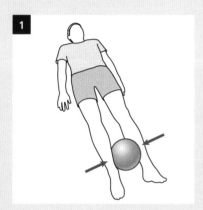

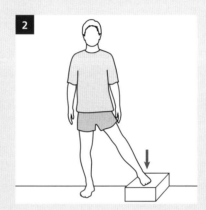

Advanced inner-thigh strengthening exercises

1. **Dynamic strengthener**. Lying on your back on the edge of a bed or bench, take your leg out over the side of the bed; keeping your knee straight and foot turned out, bring the leg up and across your other leg, then control the reverse movement; repeat 3 times, then relax completely. Build up to 10 repetitions.

2. **Dynamic-resisted strengthener**. With your ankle attached to a pulley system or band, stand with your leg held out to the side; bring your leg across in front of the other leg against the resistance, then control the reverse movement. 5–10 times.

3. **Weight-resisted strengthener**. Using an adductor machine, work through the full range of movement. 3–10 times.

4. **Inner range strengthener**. Lying on your side, with your upper leg bent behind you resting on a cushion or support, and the lower leg very slightly in front of your body with the knee straight; lift the lower leg a little way upwards, then control the reverse movement. 3–10 times.

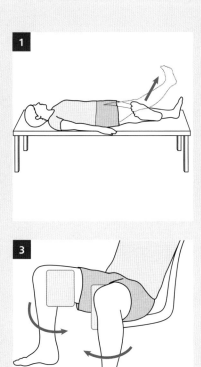

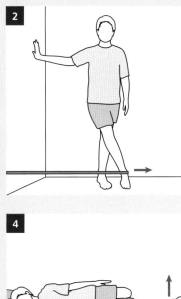

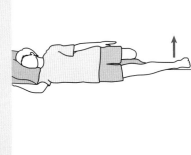

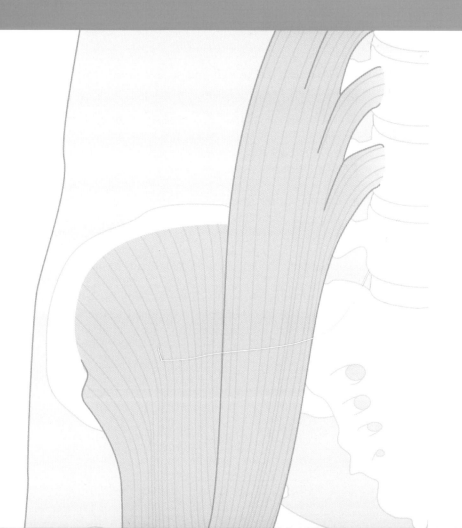

12

The Hip

RIGHT HIP SEEN FROM THE FRONT.

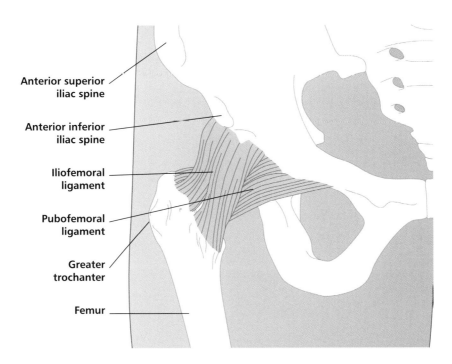

Anterior superior
iliac spine

Anterior inferior
iliac spine

Iliofemoral
ligament

Pubofemoral
ligament

Greater
trochanter

Femur

The hip joint is an extremely stable ball-and-socket joint, which links the femur to the outer side of the pelvis.

Structure

Bones

The rounded head at the top of the femur links with a shallow cup-shaped hollow called the acetabulum on the outer side of the innominate bone (hip bone). The two hip bones form the sides of the pelvic basin.

The neck of the femur connects the bone's head to its shaft. It is angled upwards and inwards, and is about 5 centimetres (2 inches) long. The top of the femur is specially constructed to withstand and transmit pressure through a kind of intricate latticework called trabeculae within the bone structure. The blood supply to the head of the femur is relatively limited, whereas the neck of the bone has a richer supply.

Capsule and ligaments

The bones of the hip joint are tightly enclosed in a fibrous capsule with a fluid-producing synovial lining. Within the capsule the bones are held with a negative pressure, which makes it very hard to pull the hip joint apart. The capsule is thickened at the front into one of the strongest ligaments in the body, the iliofemoral ligament. There are other ligaments around the joint, and a much weaker one in the centre (which many people do not even have) joining the head of the femur to the acetabulum. Bursae (fluid-filled sacs) lie under the ligaments, muscles and tendons where they cross close to each other or over a bone.

Muscles and tendons

The main muscle groups round the hip are the hip flexors, gluteals, rotators, rectus femoris and sartorius on the front of the thigh (p. 118), the hamstrings (p. 131), and the inner-thigh muscles (p. 139).

HIP FLEXORS ON THE RIGHT SIDE, SEEN FROM THE FRONT.

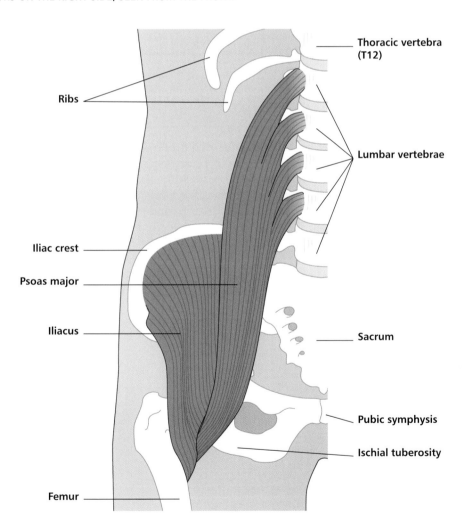

Psoas major and iliacus are the hip flexor muscles. Because they work closely together, they are often called iliopsoas, although they are separate in structure. They are deep-lying. Psoas major is attached to the front of the lumbar vertebrae in your lower back, and travels down through the pelvis to fix to a knob called the lesser trochanter on the inner side of the femur, just below the hip. Iliacus is attached to the inner surface of the innominate bone and the side of the sacrum within the pelvis, and extends downwards to blend with the psoas major tendon in a common attachment to the lesser trochanter, although some of its fibres are attached directly to the femur.

The gluteals cover the back and side of the hip. Gluteus maximus forms the rounded contour of your bottom. It is attached to the ilium, sacrum and coccyx at the back of the pelvis, and spreads down and outwards to connect with the top of the femur just below the greater trochanter and the iliotibial tract. Gluteus medius is under gluteus maximus, extending from the ilium down the back of the pelvis to the greater trochanter at the side of the femur. Gluteus minimus lies deeper still, spreading from the ilium to a point on the greater trochanter just below and in front of the attachment of gluteus medius.

The rotators are smaller than the gluteals, and consist of piriformis, obturatores externus and internus, the superior and inferior gemelli, and quadratus femoris. They connect the inner, outer and lower parts of the pelvis with the top of the femur.

How the hip works

The hip is very stable. The ball-and-socket construction allows for forward, backward, sideways and twisting movements. Acting against gravity or a resistance, with the body straight, the hip flexors combined with rectus femoris and sartorius take the leg forwards into flexion at the hip. Gluteus maximus and the hamstrings take the leg backwards into extension. Gluteus medius and gluteus minimus, with help from sartorius and tensor fasciae latae, abduct the leg, taking it outwards away from the other leg. The inner-thigh muscles bring the leg inwards, into adduction. Tensor fasciae latae and glutei medius and minimus rotate the leg inwards (medially), while the obturators, gemelli and quadratus femoris, together with gluteus maximus, piriformis, psoas major and sartorius, turn the leg outwards, into lateral rotation. Flexion and outward rotation have the greatest freedom of movement, whereas extension is limited to about 10–15 degrees.

The hip abductors, gluteus medius and gluteus minimus, act to stabilize the hips when you stand and move your legs. Those on one side contract concentrically to lift the leg, while on the opposite side they work to hold the pelvis steady. If the hip abductors are weak for any reason, standing on the weakened leg and trying to lift the other one makes the pelvis drop downwards on the moving side, so it is difficult to take a step. This is called Trendelenburg's sign.

The hip allows for a wide variety of movements, such as twisting and turning as you walk, run or dance, kicking a ball, throwing the discus or javelin, fencing, breaststroke swimming, sitting cross-legged or in lotus position, hopping and bounding in different directions, and the simple actions of touching your legs or feet. Doing the splits forwards or sideways depends on extreme mobility in the hips, pelvis and lower back. The ability to spread the legs wide apart is important for childbirth: if the mother has abnormally stiff hips, Caesarian section may be necessary for a safe delivery.

The hip is subjected to enormous pressures in the course of a lifetime. When you stand or walk, the hip transmits the weight of your trunk to your legs, under the additional pressure of gravity. When you are sitting down, the hips bear the weight of the trunk, head and arms, plus gravity, against the opposing force of the surface you sit on. When you run, jump or hop, the pressure on the hip joints increases dramatically, softened only by the efficiency with which your muscles and joints can absorb the shock.

HIP ABDUCTOR MUSCLES, ON THE RIGHT SIDE.

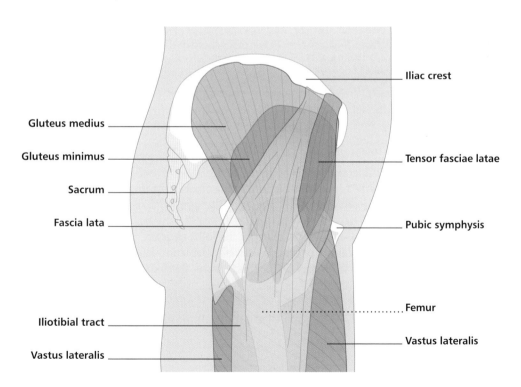

Pain and complications

Unexplained or unusual pain in the hip region may be due to an inflammatory joint condition (p. 12) or a disease such as tuberculosis. Pain can be referred to the hip region from other areas, for instance the back or pelvis.

'Irritable hip syndrome' is the name given to pain which develops in the hip for no obvious reason, causing a limp and loss of movement in the joint. All tests for hip damage or infection are apparently normal. It happens mostly in children, but can also affect adults, and the treatment is usually bed rest until the symptoms subside.

Hip region problems

The bones and soft tissues of the hip can be injured through trauma or overuse. Imbalance between the hips is often a factor, especially in overuse injuries. Pain from the hip can radiate into the groin, down the side, front or back of the thigh, and even as far as the back of the ankle. Hip injuries have a direct effect on the lower back, thigh, knee and lower leg down to the foot, and can impair shoulder function. Limping can create compensatory problems on the other side of the body.

Hip imbalance

As the hip is the link between the leg and the pelvis, it influences, and is influenced by, movements, postural patterns and abnormalities anywhere in the leg or trunk, and compensates for weakness or imbalance in either leg and on each side of the body.

Careless posture can cause imbalance between your hips, especially if you stand with your weight balanced over one leg, sit on a chair with your legs crossed at the thighs or ankles, sit with one or both legs tucked under you, or sit or stand with one foot raised on a step or support. These habits are the more harmful if you are still for long periods.

Many sports and physical activities contribute to imbalance between the hips, including javelin throwing, triple jumping, hurdling and fencing. Track running puts abnormal pressure on the left hip, because the athlete has to lean into the bends. Excessive running, especially long-distance training, can lead to overload on the hips, not only because of repetitive impact, but because the hip flexor muscles on the front of the joint shorten, and the adductor muscles along the inner thigh work harder to compensate when the front-thigh muscles get tired. When a runner with weak leg muscle, especially a child, turns the legs inwards in compensation, there is extra pressure on the hips.

Injuries in other parts of the body which cause a limp can create abnormal pressure on one or both hips.

Traumatic bone fracture

Any of the bones forming the hip can be broken or cracked in a traumatic injury. Fracture can happen at any age, but is most common in older people. Traumatic fracture can happen together with hip dislocation.

What you feel
There is usually severe pain in the groin region, but occasionally surprisingly little. The leg looks distorted. Movements at the hip are limited, painful and abnormal, and you may lose sensation in your leg. There may be bruising, swelling and bleeding. Clinical shock can set in.

Causes
Often there is a bad fall with weight applied to the bone. Fracture is more likely to happen if you have mineral deficiency or bone disease such as osteoporosis.

Directions
The injury must be treated as an emergency. You may need an operation, depending on the type of fracture and how unstable it is. One possible complication of fracture or dislocation in the hip region is avascular necrosis (p. 9), in which the head of the femur loses its blood supply and collapses. This is more likely to happen if you have underlying health problems, including kidney disease, diabetes and gout, or if you are a heavy alcohol drinker. If you notice increasing pain in the weeks following your injury, you must refer back to your practitioner urgently.

How long?
1–3 years.

Dislocation

A major traumatic injury can cause the hip joint to dislocate. The head of the femur is separated from its socket. This can happen at any age. Some children are born with congenital hip dislocation, an abnormal formation of the hip joint which is also called developmental dysplasia of the hip (DDH). This is more common in girls than boys.

What you feel
There is extreme pain, and you cannot move the joint or take weight through it. The injured leg looks visibly out of place, and is usually bruised and swollen. You are likely to feel strange sensations in your leg, or you may lose feeling altogether.

Causes
As the hip is so stable, it takes a lot of force to dislocate it. Dislocation can happen through an accident at high speed, a fall from a height, or falling with a heavy weight across the leg. The injury is more likely to happen if you have had previous hip problems, especially as a baby or in childhood, and if those problems were not treated properly at the time. Dislocation can be a complication following a total hip replacement operation.

Directions
This injury is a major emergency, and you must be taken to hospital for immediate treatment, which may involve manipulation or surgery. Babies with DDH are usually treated with special splints to help the hips develop properly, but manipulation or surgery might be needed at a later stage if the problem does not resolve.

How long?
3–12 months or longer. Babies with DDH are usually monitored over several years to prevent long-term problems.

Perthes syndrome

Following a traumatic injury, avascular necrosis can damage the rounded head of the femur, causing it to break down. This is a condition which affects young children, mainly between the ages of three and ten. It can also happen apparently spontaneously. It affects more boys than girls, but tends to be worse in girls. It usually occurs in one hip, but can be in both.

The full name of the condition is Legg-Calvé-Perthes syndrome, and it is also known as osteochondritis of the femoral head, ischaemic necrosis of the hip, and coxa plana.

What you feel
There is pain walking, which causes a limp. Movement at the hip, especially twisting, is painful and limited. Standing, kneeling and crouching down can be painful. There is usually tightness in the hip muscles, especially the adductors. Pain can be referred into the groin region or down to the knee. Sometimes the affected leg is shorter than the other.

Causes
An accident or fall can be the trigger. Other factors are thought to play a part, including blood clotting abnormality, synovitis in the hip through inflammation or infection, and exposure to passive smoking.

Directions
Exercises to keep the hip as mobile as possible are essential, and have to be continued indefinitely. If the problem develops, splinting, traction or surgery may be needed.

How long?
This is a long-term problem.

Bone stress injury

The bones of the hip, especially the upper end of the femur, can suffer a micro-crack, or stress fracture, through overuse injury. This can happen at any age, and is probably most common in adult females.

Apophysitis (damage to the growth plates of the bones) at the greater and lesser trochanters is similar to a stress fracture. It affects teenagers between the ages of 14 and 18.

What you feel
There is a gradually increasing ache over the affected area or radiating into the groin, which is usually felt after training or at night at first, but later interferes with your exercise or even walking. The pain may ease within a few days if you stop exercising, but recurs if you resume too soon.

Causes
Repetitive stress through the pull of a muscle or tendon against the bone leads to breakdown of the bone structure. Overtraining or changing a routine involving repetitive weight-bearing activities like running, jumping or dancing are the most common causes. You may have increased your training, started a new programme, or resumed after a lay-off, without allowing sufficient rest days for building up your fitness. You are more likely to suffer bone injury if you have mineral deficiency or bone disease.

Directions
You have to rest from painful activities for as long as it takes for the bone to heal completely, and do alternative exercise and fitness training to stimulate the healing. A bone scan may be needed to confirm the diagnosis. You must avoid 'trying out' your leg, as the problem will only drag on indefinitely. If you make it worse, a stress fracture can turn into a complete break. You need to have at least two weeks clear of pain after the bone has mended before making a carefully graduated return to your sport.

How long?
4–9 months.

Transient synovitis

The synovial lining of the hip becomes inflamed, suddenly or gradually. This is generally a problem in young children, mainly boys, but it can also happen to babies and adults. It is often referred to as 'irritable hip syndrome'.

What you feel
There is acute pain on all hip movements and on weight-bearing. The leg is usually held bent and turned outwards, the hip feels stiff, and walking is difficult. There may be tenderness on pressure, and pain when lying on the affected side. Pain can be referred to the groin, down the thigh, or to the knee.

Causes
Synovitis can follow a traumatic injury from a fall or jarring the joint. Often the cause is not obvious. Occasionally it is linked to a recent viral infection.

Directions
Tests should be done to make sure there is no serious underlying problem. Usually treatment consists of rest from painful activities. If the problem gets worse, or a high temperature develops, you should refer back to your practitioner urgently.

How long?
10 days, sometimes longer.

Slipped capital femoral epiphysis

The growth area (growth plate) just below the head of the femur breaks, so the bone parts slide on each other. This can happen in one hip or both, and is more common in males than females. It is mainly a teenage problem, but can happen to pre-teens.

What you feel
In rare cases the pain comes on suddenly and very severely. More often it occurs gradually in the hip, groin and/or knee, especially on walking. All hip movements become difficult and limited. The leg may be shortened, and held with the foot turned out.

Causes
The reason for the slipped epiphysis is not known. It is often associated with being overweight. Sometimes it follows a minor injury which has caused a limp.

Directions
An acute slip is usually treated as an emergency, as the pain is so severe. In all cases you have to avoid taking weight through the leg. Your doctor or specialist may recommend rest in bed. If overpronation of the foot is a factor, corrective orthotics may be recommended. Most often surgery is needed to stabilize the bone parts and prevent complications such as avascular necrosis or osteoarthritis.

How long?
This is a long-term problem. Follow-up by the specialist usually extends over at least two years.

'Snapping hip'

Tightness or thickening of one or more of the hip tendons, coupled with inflammation or enlargement of a bursa, can cause a snapping sound when the hip is moved. Snapping can also be caused by damage to soft tissues inside the joint. This may be felt to the side or front of the joint, or deep inside. It is an overuse problem which can happen at any age, but is most common in the late teens and young adulthood.

What you feel
The snapping noise happens when you move the hip forwards and backwards, or straighten your leg after it has been bent for a while. Pain varies according to which tissues are involved.

Causes
Intensive training in activities like running, horse riding, gymnastics, football, baseball, weightlifting, powerlifting and ballet can cause attritional damage to the soft tissues round the hip. The problem is more likely to happen if you have mechanical imbalance such as a longer leg on one side (p. 171), weakness in any of the hip or pelvic muscle groups, or poor foot movements, especially overpronation (p. 43).

Directions
Rest from painful activities and a rehabilitation programme are usually sufficient, but in a chronic case you may be offered an injection or surgery. Orthotics may help if faulty foot mechanics have contributed.

How long?
2 weeks to several months.

Bursitis

Inflammation in one or more of the bursae around the hip causes a localized point of pain. It is most common at the side of the hip (trochanteric bursitis) or at the front (iliopsoas bursitis). This is usually an overuse injury, but is sometimes caused by trauma. It can affect anyone, but is most common in adult females.

What you feel
There is pain over the affected bursa when there is pressure on it, especially if you lie on that side at night, or run on hilly ground. The leg may get stiff if you sit still for long periods.

Causes
Overtraining in sports like running and cycling can cause irritation. A fall on to the hip can cause deep bruising, leading to inflammation. The problem is more likely to happen if you have mechanical imbalance in the leg, especially leg length differences (p. 171).

Directions
Any contributory factors should be corrected. You may be offered an injection.

How long?
2 weeks to several months.

Hip muscle and tendon injury

Any of the muscles or tendons round the hip can be torn, partly torn or strained through trauma or overuse. Injury can happen at any age.

What you feel
There is pain when the injured muscles are activated, especially against a load or resistance, and when they are stretched. The pain may make you limp. There may be visible bruising or swelling in the area.

Causes
Trauma can be caused by a blocked movement, as in catching your foot as you run or jump in any direction, a mistimed kick in tae kwon do, or a blocked tackle in football. Overtraining in sports which stress the hip muscles, such as running, fencing, soccer, cycling and horse riding can lead to overuse strains. Injury is more likely to happen if you have imbalance around your hips, or if you have had previous leg injuries. Sometimes faulty foot mechanics contribute.

Directions
Any contributory factors should be corrected: orthotics can help if foot mechanics are involved.

How long?
2 weeks to 3 months.

Osteoarthritis (osteoarthrosis)

The hip joint can suffer from wear-and-tear damage or degenerative arthritis. The cartilage surface of the bone ends wears thin and can become pitted. Sometimes bony spurs form where muscle attachments lie close to the joint. It is usually a problem from late middle age onwards, but can happen as early as the late twenties.

What you feel
In the early stages there may be an ache or stiffness, which you feel after exercise, or after being still for some time. There is usually pain at night. The pain gradually gets worse, and can affect your walking, making you limp. You may feel it mainly in the groin, but it can affect all sides of the hip region. Joint movement becomes increasingly restricted. A severely arthritic hip can become fixed in the flexed and internally rotated position, although in some cases it turns outwards.

Causes
Many factors contribute to hip degeneration. It is associated with overtraining in sports which cause repetitive jarring and compression on the joint. If joint movement is limited by tightness in any of the hip muscles, especially the hip flexors, part of the femoral head will be subjected to extra wear. Problems can arise just as much from the forced turnout position classical ballerinas adopt from an early age as from a sedentary job in which you keep your hips bent for hours on end. Hip imbalance which develops in the late teens can cause early onset osteoarthritis, as can childhood hip problems if not properly treated. Some people have a hereditary family tendency to osteoarthritis.

Directions
Even when severe degeneration in a hip is evident on an X-ray or scan, it is not necessarily painful, if you keep the joint functional. You should maintain a regular regime of protective exercises, and avoid activities which place undue stress on the hips. If the pain develops to an unbearable stage, you may be offered surgery to replace part or all of the damaged joint.

How long?
This is a long-term condition.

The Hip

Rehabilitation and recovery

Acute phase

You should use the circulatory care measures (p. 27), according to your practitioner's instructions. You may be treated with electrical muscle stimulation for the vastus medialis obliquus (p. 112), to help restore basic strength to your leg and reduce pressure on the hip. As soon as possible, you should start alternative training (p. 25), using mainly your arms and shoulders.

Early phase

Crutches are used in the early stages of recovery after any significant hip problem. Your practitioner will tell you when you can do early stage exercises to help you to walk correctly (p. 34), and when you can start the basic hip mobilizing and strengthening exercises. If possible, these should be combined with straight-leg raises (p. 115) and the basic stretching and strengthening exercises for the front thigh (pp. 126–127), hamstrings (pp. 135–136), inner thigh (pp. 144–145) and abdominals (pp. 190–191). Aim at two or three sessions each day. You should perform the exercises on both sides, if possible, but with more repetitions on the injured side.

Recovery phase

In the later stages you will need to work on balance exercises (p. 36) and the advanced exercises for correct walking (p. 38). As you regain strength and mobility in the joint, the advanced hip mobilizing, stretching and strengthening exercises should be combined with those for the calf (p. 82), knee (p. 113), front thigh (p. 128), hamstrings (p. 137), inner thigh (p. 146), pelvis (pp. 182–183), back (pp. 236–238) and shoulder (pp. 264–266). Add gradually increasing weights or resistance for the strengthening exercises when possible.

You should be able to take your weight comfortably on the injured leg, and to squat fully, before progressing to the final recovery phase (p. 308).

Re-injury prevention

For long-term protection of the hips, you should always take care of your posture, and maintain a regular exercise programme for hip mobility and muscle strength.

Basic hip mobilizing exercises

The first three exercises are best done on a smooth surface, perhaps using talcum powder on a polished board to help the gliding movement.

1. **Foot rotation, lying.** Lying on your back with your legs relaxed, straight and apart, rotate your feet gently, making circles clockwise, then anticlockwise. 10–20 times.
2. **Hip and knee flexion, lying.** Lying on your back with your legs straight, slide your foot towards your bottom gently, then straighten the leg out again. 5–10 times in quick succession.
3. **Hip abduction, lying.** Lying on your back, slide your leg out sideways as far as is comfortable, then bring it back to centre rhythmically. 5–10 times.
4. **Hip rotation, lying.** Lying on your back with your feet apart, turn your feet and legs outwards as far as you can, then inwards. 10–20 times.

5. **Hip flexion and extension, standing**. Standing up straight, swing one leg gently forwards and backwards, rhythmically. 10–20 times.

6. **Hip abduction and adduction, standing**. Standing up straight, swing one leg out sideways then across in front of your body, keeping the knee straight. 10–20 times.

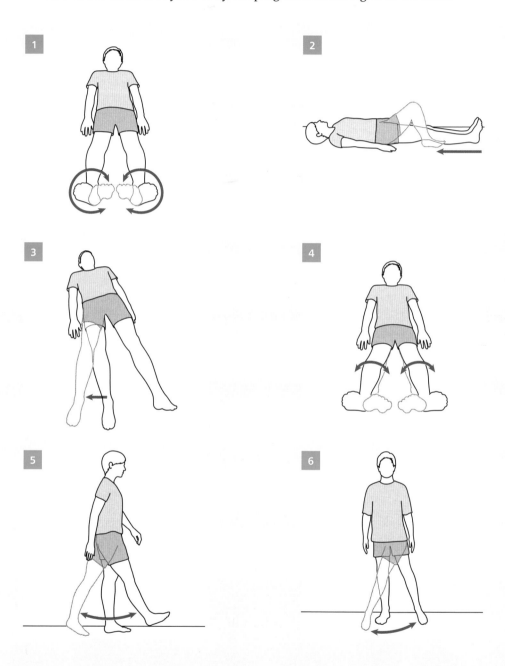

Basic hip strengthening exercises

1. **Hip extension, stomach-lying**. Lying on your stomach, tighten your buttock muscles, lock your knee straight and lift the leg up a little way behind you; hold for a count of 2, then lower the leg and relax completely. 5–10 times.

2. **Hip flexion and extension, standing**. Standing on your uninjured leg, take the other leg forwards and hold for a count of 2; take it backwards behind you a little way, and again hold for a count of 2, then relax. 5–10 times.

3. **Hip abduction, side-lying**. Lying on your side, injured leg uppermost, with a pillow between your knees, lift your upper leg a little way, keeping your hip well forward and your knee locked straight; hold for a count of 2, then slowly lower. 5–10 times.

4. **Hip flexion and abduction, lying**. Lying on your back, lift your leg up a little way, take it out sideways, back to centre and slowly lower it, keeping your knee locked straight throughout. 5–10 times.

5. **Hip extension and abduction, stomach-lying**. Lying on your stomach, lift one leg up behind you a little way, take it out sideways, keeping the knee locked straight; slowly reverse the movement. 5–10 times.

6. **Hip raise, crook-lying**. Lying on your back, with a pillow under your head, knees bent and arms alongside you; breathing normally, lift your hips up a little way, hold for a count of 2, then slowly lower your hips and relax completely. 5–10 times.

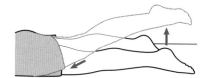

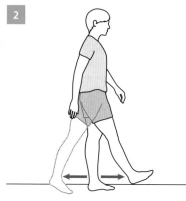

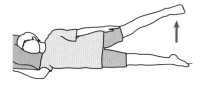

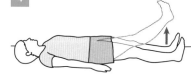

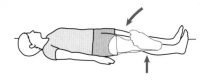

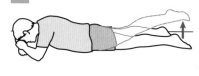

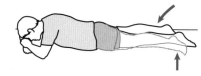

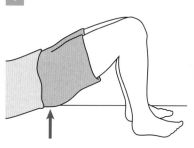

Advanced hip stretching and mobilizing

1. **Front-hip stretch, stomach-lying**. Lying on your stomach and place your hands under your shoulders, palms facing down and fingers forwards; straighten your elbows as far as you can, keeping your hips down and your head up; hold for a count of 6, then relax. 5–10 times.

2. **Front-hip mobilizer, lying**. Lying on your back at the edge of a high bench, take your leg downwards over the side; keeping your knee bent, lift and lower the leg in a rhythmical motion. 10–20 times.

3. **Inner-thigh mobilizer, sitting**. Sitting on the floor, bend your knees to place the soles of your feet together; take your knees outwards in a little bouncing movement. 10–20 times using your muscles only, then 10–20 times pressing the knees gently with your hands.

4. **Rotation mobilizer, stomach-lying**. Lying on your stomach with your knees slightly apart and bent to right angles, take your feet outwards and inwards in a rhythmical motion, keeping the pelvis still, so that your hips twist inwards and outwards. 10–20 times.

5. **Hip abductor stretch, lying**. Lying on your back with one leg straight, the other bent up and crossed over the straight leg, with the foot placed at the outer side of the straight knee, gently push your upper knee sideways over the other leg with your hand, until you feel a slight stretching sensation over the outer side of the hip and thigh; hold the position for a count of 6, then relax. 3–10 times.

6. **Hip abductor stretch, sitting**. Sitting on the floor with one leg straight, the other bent with the foot placed on the outer side of the straight leg, twist your trunk so that you can place the opposite arm on the outer side of the bent knee; gently press your arm against your leg while keeping your trunk turned away from your legs; hold for a count of 6, then relax. 3–10 times.

7. **Gluteal stretch, sitting**. Sitting on an upright chair or bench, lean forwards as far as you can; hold the position for a count of 6, then relax. 3–10 times.

8. **Complex hip mobilizer, lying**. Lying on your back on the end of a high bench, with your thighs supported and your legs over the end, bend one knee, and bring it towards your chest with your hands; pull the knee into your chest 3 times, keeping your other leg down. 3–10 times.

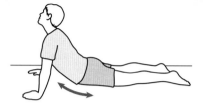

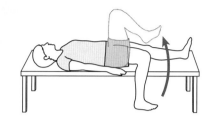
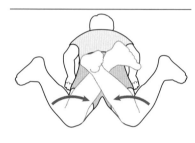

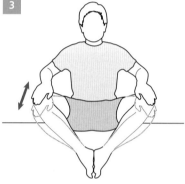

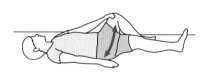

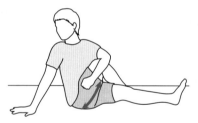
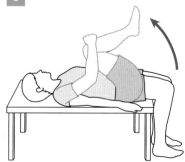

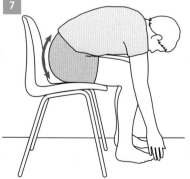

Advanced hip strengthening exercises

1. **Complex abductor strengthener**. Lying on one side, bend the upper hip and knee to right angles; keeping the leg bent, lift the knee upwards away from your body and lower it 3–5 times, then relax. 5–10 times.

2. **Hip circling, lying**. Lying on your back on the edge of a bed, lift your leg up and draw clockwise circles in the air with your foot, keeping your knee locked straight; start with small circles, then make them as large as possible. 3–20 times.

3. **Side-raise, on bent arm**. Lying on your side, with your body straight, rest on your elbow and forearm; lift your hips upwards so that you balance on your forearm and the side of your foot; hold for a count of 2, then slowly lower your hips. 5–10 times.

4. **Hip abduction, standing**. Standing up straight with your arms by your sides, lift one leg straight out sideways and lower it 3–5 times without putting the foot down; repeat with the other leg, then relax completely. 5–10 times.

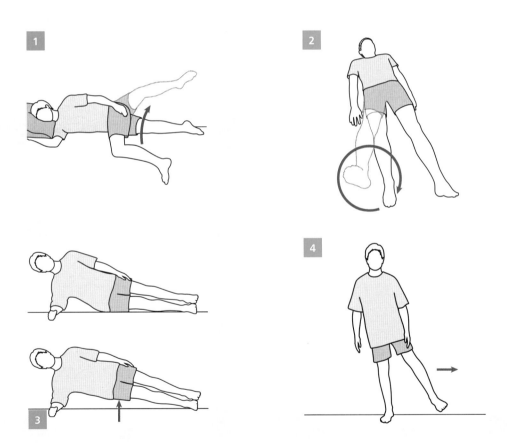

13

The Pelvis

FRONT VIEW OF PELVIS.

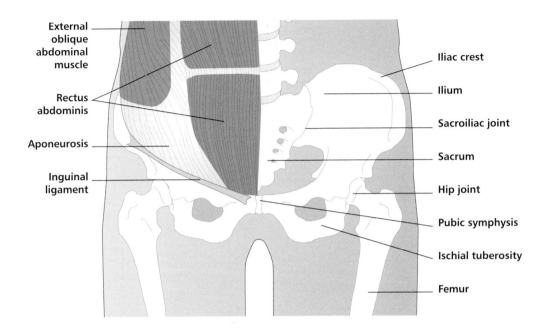

External oblique abdominal muscle

Rectus abdominis

Aponeurosis

Inguinal ligament

Iliac crest

Ilium

Sacroiliac joint

Sacrum

Hip joint

Pubic symphysis

Ischial tuberosity

Femur

The pelvis is the link between your legs and trunk or torso. Adult females have a wider pelvis than males.

Structure

The pelvis is shaped like a basin, with the two innominate bones (hip bones) at the sides and front, and the sacrum at the back. The bones are linked together by soft tissues including ligaments and muscles.

Bones

Each innominate bone consists of a flat part called the ilium, which forms your flank. At its lower part, the innominate bone turns into struts comprising the pubis in front, and the ischium behind. The three parts join at the acetabulum, the hollowed cup of the hip joint. The ilium is topped by a curved ridge called the iliac crest, which you can feel with your hands, just below your waist. The main part or body of the pubis is at the front. The upper strut of the pubis, which leads from its body to the front of the acetabulum, is called the superior pubic ramus (branch), while the lower one, leading to the ischium, is the inferior pubic ramus. The main part of the ischium lies at the lower part of the acetabulum, and forms a strut called the ischial ramus, which curves to join the inferior pubic ramus. The rami form a ring, and the gap in the centre is called the obturator foramen. The ischial tuberosity is the under part of the bone where it bends to turn upwards and forwards to meet the pubic ramus. This is your seat bone, which you can feel with your hand if you press directly under your buttock when you are sitting down.

The sacrum is a wedge-shaped bone which forms the lowest part of the spinal column, and ends in the tiny coccyx, or tail bone. You can feel the sacrum and coccyx with your hand, under the skin in the lowest part of your back.

Joints and ligaments

The pubic symphysis is the joint where the two pubic bones from either side of the body meet in the midline at the front of the pelvis. It is a fibrocartilaginous joint, so it is not lubricated by synovial fluid, and is held together by strong ligaments and a fibrous disc. The sacroiliac joint, the junction between the sacrum and the innominate bone, is synovial. It is usually called a plane joint, although its surfaces are irregular rather than flat. It is held together by strong ligaments, which are arranged horizontally, vertically and diagonally. You can feel the joint where it forms dimples on either side of the midline just above the buttocks.

The inguinal ligament is a thick, strong band formed from the fibrous covering of the external oblique abdominal muscle in the lower part of the abdominal region. It is attached to the anterior inferior iliac spine on the front of the innominate bone, and extends downwards to fix on to the top of the pubic bone. The inguinal canal, which lies slightly in front of the inguinal ligament, provides a protected passageway from the abdominal region to the top of the thigh for blood vessels and nerves. Just behind the inguinal ligament is the femoral canal, a passageway for lymph vessels, which ends in the femoral ring at the top of the thigh.

Muscles

The lower part of the pelvis contains the pelvic floor muscles, which control your private parts. The main muscles which create movement and stability in the pelvic structure are the abdominals (p. 185), back extensors (p. 214), hamstrings (p. 131), adductors (p. 139) and hip muscles (p. 149).

Functions

The pelvis protects the abdominal contents, and buffers or transmits loading between the trunk and the legs. When you stand upright, the line of gravity in the body (p. 216) generally passes in front of the sacrum. The body's centre of gravity varies according to a number of factors, but is usually considered to be in front of the second sacral segment (two down from the end of the lumbar vertebrae).

The pelvis is a very stable structure: the symphysis pubis allows very little, if any, movement, while the sacroiliac joints permit a small degree of gliding or shearing. During late pregnancy and childbirth, the pelvic joints give a little to allow more space.

The pelvic basin moves as a whole: it tilts forwards and backwards when both sides work together. When you tighten your abdominal muscles, pulling them in and curving your back, your pelvis tilts backwards. If you arch your back to hollow the lumbar curve, your back muscles tighten to tilt your pelvis forwards. These movements are a major part of the butterfly swimming stroke. On a racing bicycle and galloping horse, the rider's pelvis is held in backward tilt. In dressage horse riding the more the rider's back is straight and the legs extended, the more the pelvis is tilted forwards.

Movements on one side of the pelvis involve combined action by the abdominals and back muscles on that side. When a movement happens on one side of the pelvis, the opposite takes place on the other: if you stand straight and hitch one leg upwards, keeping it parallel to the other leg, the opposite side of the pelvis tips downwards. Complex one-sided movements such as kicking a ball or throwing a javelin involve the sacroiliac joints: the slight shearing or rotatory movement on one side is usually balanced by the opposite motion on the other side.

Your pelvis is affected by the balance between the muscles around your pelvis and lower back, and by your postural habits as you go through the processes of growing and aging. The sacroiliac joints tend to stiffen with age to become fibrosed or ossified, a process which starts sooner in males, and most often after the menopause in females.

Pain and complications

Unusual or unexplained pain in the pelvis can be due to inflammatory joint conditions or internal problems affecting the urinary, digestive or reproductive systems. Hormonal changes in females due to pregnancy, the menstrual cycle, menopause, the contraceptive pill or hormone replacement therapy can be a factor in pain in the sacroiliac region at the back of the pelvis. In both males and females pain can also be referred from your back or hip, without necessarily causing pain at its source.

Ankylosing spondylitis

Of the inflammatory conditions which can cause intermittent, apparently arbitrary pain, ankylosing spondylitis is one which tends to affect the sacroiliac joints specifically. It is a progressive condition which can run in families. It mainly affects teenage boys, and the condition is often misdiagnosed as overuse injury. The first sign is usually morning stiffness in one or both sacroiliac joints, often accompanied or preceded by plantar fasciitis (p. 49). If it develops, the stiffness and pain can spread from the sacroiliac joints and hips up the spine and into the shoulders and elbows. Eventually, the joints can lock up completely, causing severe limitation of movement.

The most effective treatment for ankylosing spondylitis is a comprehensive exercise programme to maintain full joint mobility together with muscle strength and flexibility. Exercises have a dramatic effect in improving function and reducing pain, even in patients who have suffered the condition for years.

Pelvic injuries

The bones, joints and soft tissues in the pelvis can be injured through trauma or overuse at any age. Pelvic region injuries have a direct effect on the hips and lower back, and can disrupt shoulder and leg activity.

Short leg syndrome

Most people have different leg lengths, known technically as leg length discrepancy. This does not necessarily cause problems, but it can contribute to pain in the lower back, pelvis or hips, and other areas, including the feet. There are two types of discrepancy: real and apparent shortening. In real shortening the leg bones are of different lengths, while in apparent shortening the bones are reasonably equal, but a difference is created because the pelvis and back tilt sideways.

What you feel
When leg length discrepancy is a factor, your back, hip or pelvic region pain is worse when you are on your feet, standing, walking or running, than when you are sitting down.

Causes
Unequal leg lengths may be present at birth. Both types can develop through compensatory mechanisms following leg or back injury, or due to poor postural habits, like standing with your weight over one leg or sitting with your legs crossed or curled under you. Running bends on the track or distance running on a camber can create discrepancy if you do not vary your training.

Directions
Your practitioner will take some measurements to verify whether you have short leg syndrome. There are different ways of measuring. Usually measurements are taken on each side to the inner edge of your ankle bone (medial malleolus) from the top edge of your greater trochanter at the hip, from the anterior superior iliac spine on the front top edge of your innominate bone, from the umbilicus and/or from the xiphoid process at the lowest tip of the sternum (breastbone).

If you have significant shortening of one leg, you will be recommended to use a heel lift or custom-made orthotic, or to build up the shoe on that side in the case of real or long-standing discrepancy.

In either case you will be given exercises to correct muscle imbalance, which you should continue indefinitely.

How long?
A foot lift can make a difference within the first few days. Correcting muscle imbalance and postural habits takes several months.

The Pelvis

Traumatic bone fracture

Any of the bones of the pelvis can be cracked or broken through trauma, which can happen at any age. In a stable fracture the bone parts remain close together and in line, whereas they move and become deformed if the fracture is unstable.

Avulsion fracture, in which the bony attachment point of a muscle or tendon breaks off, can happen in the pelvic bones. It is particularly common in teenagers, but can happen at any age.

What you feel
A major fracture is extremely painful, and usually causes bleeding, bruising and swelling. You cannot stand up or walk. There may also be damage to internal organs and nerves, causing a wide variety of symptoms, including losing control of passing urine or of your bowel motions. The accident can lead to shock.

An avulsion fracture is less dramatic. There is usually acute pain when it happens. There may or may not be bleeding. Later you feel pain over the injured area on movements or direct pressure, often with bruising and some swelling.

Causes
A major injury involves a serious accident, such as a fall under load. The pelvis can also be fractured by a direct blow. When this happens over the iliac crest, it is called a 'hip pointer', a term which is also used for deep bruising on the bone. Pelvic fractures happen more easily if your bones are weakened by mineral deficiency or disease such as osteoporosis.

An avulsion fracture can be caused when a muscle is blocked as it contracts. This can happen along the iliac crest as you twist your body forcefully, for instance in tae kwon do: the lower attachments of the abdominal oblique muscles can pull the bone apart. The hamstrings can pull off their attachment point on the ischium if you mistime a kick, or fall with your leg straight out in front of you.

Directions
A major traumatic fracture must be treated as an emergency, and may need surgery. Stable traumatic and avulsion fractures are usually treated with rest, followed by gradual rehabilitation of the trunk and leg muscles. You will need crutches at first.

How long?
Major injury: up to 2 years.
Uncomplicated stable fracture: 6–12 months.
Avulsion fracture: 3–6 months.

Bone stress injuries

A stress fracture is an overuse injury which causes micro-damage or cracking in the hard substance of a bone. It can happen in any of the pelvic bones, especially the pubic rami and the sacrum. It can happen at any age. It is probably most prevalent in young and middle-aged females, and least common in very young children.

Apophysitis is an overuse injury in which the growth plates of the bones are damaged. This can happen in many areas of the pelvis, notably the iliac crest, the superior and inferior iliac spines, the pubic symphysis and the ischial tuberosity. Teenagers between 14 and 18 are the main sufferers.

What you feel
There is a gradually increasing ache over the affected bone, felt at first after exercising or at night, and later on during exercise. If the problem is allowed to develop, walking can hurt. The pain eases with a few days' rest, but recurs with increasing force if you try to resume your normal training too soon.

Causes
Consistent repetitive pressure by a muscle or tendon against a bone causes the damage. It is always associated with a change of routine, an increase in repetitive training, insufficient rest days after repetitive routines, and failure to do conditioning training. It is a particular risk of long-distance running when you initially take up the sport, increase your training mileage, or resume training after a lay-off. It is more likely to happen if you have mineral deficiency or bone disease.

Directions
The stress fracture is diagnosed through the history of your pain and activities, and, if necessary a bone scan, as stress fractures usually fail to show up on X-rays until they are healing. You have to stop doing the activity which caused the problem for long enough to allow the bone(s) to heal completely. You must do alternative exercise and training to stimulate healing. You should not restart training until you have had at least two weeks without pain after the bone has healed. Repetitive training has to be resumed in easy stages, and you should maintain an alternative conditioning programme indefinitely.

How long?
2–6 months.

Hernia

In tissues which separate one compartment of the body from another, such as the abdominal area and the top of the thigh, there are openings to allow blood vessels and nerves to pass through. If the opening becomes enlarged for any reason, the contents of a compartment may start to press through the space to appear on the wrong side of the containing tissues. This is called a hernia. If the herniated material becomes trapped and cut off from its blood supply, it is called a strangulated hernia.

In the groin region a hernia which occurs through the inguinal canal is called an inguinal hernia, while a hernia through the femoral ring is called a femoral hernia.

A hernia can occur at any age, and is more common in males than females.

What you feel
A visible lump appears in the groin, which may or may not be painless, and tends to come and go. Pain may develop and gradually get worse. You may have pain if you cough or sneeze, or on certain leg movements. If the hernia becomes strangulated, it is usually extremely painful.

Causes
Increased pressure in the abdominal area is the major cause. This can result from lifting or carrying heavy weights, especially if you lift incorrectly (p. 216); coughing and sneezing without bracing your back; and doing isometric exercises for the stomach muscles, especially double-leg raises lying on your back.

In very young children a hernia can be the result of a defect at birth. Congenital defects can also be a factor in hernia at a later stage.

Directions
A strangulated hernia should be treated as an emergency. For the more minor version, if it is causing problems, you may need surgery. There are different types of hernia repair to choose from.

How long?
If you have an operation, your surgeon will spell out the phases of your recovery. In general, you have to take it easy for at least six weeks, gently regaining full movement and strength in the hip and abdominal regions. Strenuous exercise, lifting weights or carrying loads must be avoided for at least six months or more, according to your surgeon's instructions. Isometric abdominal exercises like the double-leg raise should be excluded altogether.

Gilmore's groin

Trauma or overuse can cause a strain or tear in the lower edge of the oblique abdominal muscles together with related tendons and soft tissues in the groin area. It can seem like a hernia, but usually no hernia is present. It can happen at any age, and is more common in males than females.

What you feel
There is pain in the groin region which is felt after training involving running or kicking. The pain increases if you continue training, and you feel it whenever you turn your body. Coughing and sneezing may also hurt.

Causes
A blocked kick or tackle in football, or a twisting fall at full stretch, can cause a traumatic strain or tear. Overuse injury can result from repetitive kicking training for karate, rugby or football, or from forceful trunk twisting movements, as in tennis serving or throwing the javelin.

Directions
A strengthening programme is essential. If the problem is persistent, you may be offered an operation.

How long?
6–12 weeks, sometimes longer.

Groin friction

Persistent pressure on the groin can cause damage to the skin and its underlying structures, especially the nerve systems. It can happen at any age, but is most common in adult males.

What you feel
You may feel pain, numbness, tingling or itching sensations. The skin in the groin can become inflamed, damaged or infected. Sometimes males suffer an extremely uncomfortable constant erection, a condition called priapism.

Causes
In cyclists the problem is usually caused by the saddle, which may be the wrong shape or size for the individual. Tight shorts or underpants, especially of synthetic materials, can cause friction problems in runners.

Directions
Identify and correct the cause of the problem, if possible. Refer to your doctor if you have signs of infection, or if the symptoms persist.

How long?
2 weeks to several months.

Meralgia paraesthetica (Bernhardt-Roth syndrome)

The lateral cutaneous nerve of the thigh becomes damaged, trapped or compressed, usually in its pathway near the attachment point of the inguinal ligament on the front of the ilium. This is commonly an overuse problem, which happens mainly in adults.

What you feel
Pain is referred in the nerve pathway along the outer side of the thigh down to the knee. The outer thigh can also become hypersensitive or numb, and there may be tingling sensations. The pain is not directly related to specific movements. Standing still for long periods or wearing tight clothing round your waist, lower abdomen, hip or groin can make the pain worse. In children the pain can be intense, hindering activity.

Causes
The trapped nerve syndrome can follow overuse injury in the lower abdomen, such as inguinal ligament damage, or a strain or tear in the lower end of the abdominal muscles. Injury can happen through repetitive activities like long-distance running or cycling, especially if you wear tight underwear or shorts or have gained weight. Body armour that fits too tightly in the lower abdomen or groin can cause the problem in martial arts players.

Directions
Do not wear tight clothing over the groin or abdominal regions. You may need to lose weight and strengthen and stretch your abdominal muscles. If your pain persists, you may be offered nerve-block injections or, as a last resort, surgery.

How long?
3–9 months.

Osteitis pubis

Inflammation in the pubic symphysis at the front of the pelvic basin can happen as an overuse injury, and occasionally through trauma. It is most common in males.

What you feel
There is an ache or pain over the pubic symphysis on running or strenuous abdominal exercises. The pain sometimes spreads along the groin region or up to the lower part of the abdomen. It eases with rest. The area feels tender on pressure.

Causes
Trauma can be caused by a blocked movement, as in catching your foot as you run or jump in Overtraining or sudden overstretching in sports like field or ice hockey, soccer and American football can cause the problem. Osteitis pubis can be a complication of pregnancy or following an operation in the groin region.

Directions
Usually rest from painful activities is sufficient, coupled with rehabilitation exercises. Sometimes surgery is needed.

How long?
3–24 months.

Sacroiliac injuries

The sacroiliac joints can be strained, singly or together, through sudden or repetitive bending and twisting stresses. Injury can happen at any age, but is least common in children. Sacroiliac joint injury often happens in conjunction with problems in the hip region and lumbar spine.

What you feel
There is pain on one or both sides in the lowest part of the back. Sometimes the pain radiates to about halfway down the back of the thigh. Pain is felt on movements of the trunk and legs, including bending backwards and sideways; bending forwards to a certain angle, usually about 30 degrees from the upright position; and bending forwards slightly and turning to one side. Sitting still, especially with your legs stretched out or tucked under you, or lying flat on your back or stomach can also bring on discomfort and stiffness.

Causes
Bending forward and twisting can put a shearing stress on the sacroiliac joints, so risk sports include tennis, fencing, hurdling and javelin throwing. Overstriding while running or hurdling, overtraining for bend running on the track, jarring the lead leg in cricket bowling or mistiming a kick in soccer can all cause adverse pressure on the joints.

You are more vulnerable if you have muscle or joint imbalance in the hips and trunk, leg length discrepancy, or uneven foot mechanics. Females are more prone to sacroiliac injury at certain phases of the menstrual cycle, especially just before a period, during pregnancy, immediately after giving birth, and during the menopause. Hormone replacement therapy is sometimes a factor.

Directions
Try to avoid activities and positions which cause pain. In a severe case you may be advised to lie down for a few days until the acute pain has passed. If lying flat is uncomfortable, lie on your back with your knees supported on pillows, or on your front with a pillow under your stomach. Sometimes a back support can help limit the pain. Treatments aim to relieve the symptoms, and include manual therapy and sometimes injection. After the acute phase, exercises to restore muscle balance are essential.

How long?
10 days to several months.

Coccyx injuries

The tail bone can be fractured, displaced or bruised at any age through trauma, and, less commonly, through overuse stress.

What you feel
There is severe to agonizing pain on direct pressure on the coccyx, especially when you sit on a hard surface. In some cases pain is present all the time. If nerves have been damaged as well as the bone, you may experience tingling or numbness. Bowel movements are usually painful.

Causes
Coccyx injury is often caused by a fall on to the bone. It can be a cumulative injury, for instance through intensive horse riding. Sometimes trauma happens as a mother gives birth.

Directions
You may need to use a hollowed-out cushion or a rubber ring in order to sit comfortably. Rest can be sufficient for the problem to subside, but, if not, you may need manipulation, or, as a last resort, surgery.

How long?
6 weeks to many months.

Rehabilitation and recovery

Acute phase
You should use the circulatory care measures (p. 27) according to your practitioner's instructions.

Early phase
As you recover, you will work on early progressive weight-bearing (p. 34) and balance exercises (p. 36) according to your practitioner's instructions. Within pain limits you might do the basic mobility and strengthening exercises, which may be combined with the essential VMO exercises (p. 112), straight-leg raises (p. 115) and basic mobilizing and strengthening exercises for the front thigh (pp. 126–127), hamstrings (pp. 135–136), inner thigh (pp. 144–145), hip (pp. 160–163), lower back (pp. 230–234), abdominals (pp. 190–191) and shoulders (pp. 258–260), according to your situation. Aim to do one to three sessions a day. Alternative training for the unaffected parts of your body should start as soon as possible (p. 25).

Recovery phase
You should progress to the advanced exercises for correct walking (p. 38), as well as the advanced mobilizing and strengthening exercises for the pelvis, hips and all related areas. Before going on to the final recovery phase (p. 308), you must regain full flexibility and strength in the abdominal region, as well as stability and balance in the hips.

The Pelvis

Basic pelvic mobilizing exercises

1. **Pelvic tilt, crook-lying**. Lying on your back with your knees bent and slightly apart, tighten your stomach muscles and press your lower back into the floor to tilt your pelvis backwards, then arch your back away from the floor, tilting the pelvis forwards. 10–20 times.

2. **Pelvic tilt, sitting or standing**. Sitting or standing upright, gently tilt your pelvis to hollow and curve your lower back. 10–20 times.

3. **Simple lower back rotation**. Lying on your back with your knees bent and legs together, gently swing your knees from side to side as far as you can, keeping your feet and lower back in contact with the floor. 10–20 times.

4. **Sitting pelvic rotation**. Sitting on a chair or stool, gently transfer your body weight in a circular motion over your hips, keeping your shoulders level: as your weight shifts backwards, your back curves and your stomach should be hollow; forwards, your back arches to press your stomach to the front; sideways, your trunk elongates on the weight-bearing side. 10–20 times clockwise, then anticlockwise.

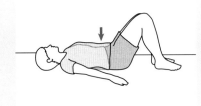

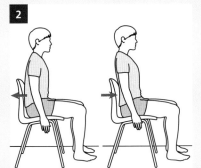

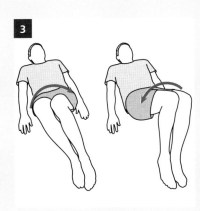

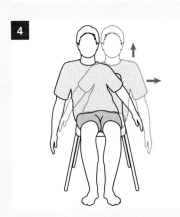

Basic pelvic strengthening exercises

1. **Pelvic floor isometric exercise**. Sitting, standing or lying down, tighten your pelvic floor muscles as though you were trying to prevent yourself from passing urine; hold the contraction for a count of 5, then relax. 3–6 times.

2. **Isometric gluteal contraction**. Lying on your back or stomach, tighten your buttock muscles; hold the contraction for a count of 5, then relax. 3–6 times.

3. **Hip flexion, crook-lying**. Lying on your back with your knees bent, lift one leg up towards your chest, keeping the knee bent; slowly reverse the movement. 5–10 times.

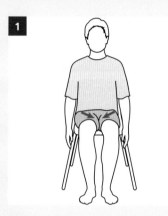

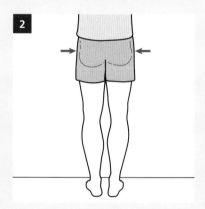

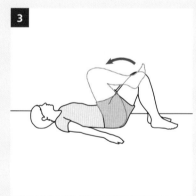

Advanced pelvic mobilizing exercises

1. **Four-point mobilizer**. On your hands and knees, stretch one leg out sideways with your knee straight, foot on the floor, and turn your head to look at your foot, keeping your head in line with your trunk; swing your foot round behind you, and turn your head to look at your foot; repeat 3–5 times in quick succession on one side, then the other. 5–10 times overall.

2. **Flexion-extension mobilizer**. On your hands and knees, bend your head down and bend one knee up to touch your knee to your forehead; take the leg backwards as you lift your head upwards. 5–10 times on one side then the other.

3. **Advanced lower back rotation**. Lying on your back with your arms stretched out sideways at right angles to your body, lift one leg up in the air as far as you can, with the knee straight, and take it over the other leg towards the opposite hand to stretch your lower back area, keeping your upper body as still as possible. 5–10 times on one side, then the other.

4. **Extensor muscle release**. Lying on your back, bend your knees up to your chest, put your arms round your legs just below the knees and clasp your hands together; press your legs against your hands, blocking any movement; hold for a count of 2; repeat 3 times, and relax completely; then gently pull your legs in towards your chest with your hands to stretch the gluteal muscles and lower back. 3–5 times.

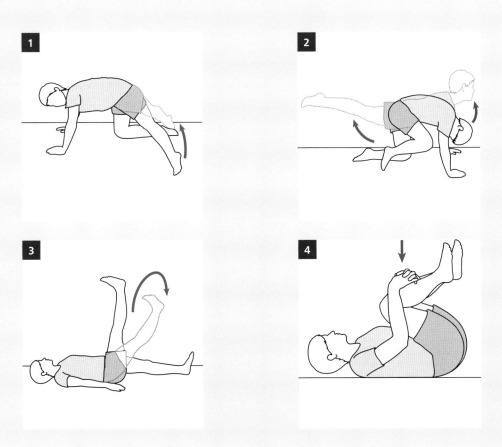

Advanced pelvic strengthening exercises

1. **Hip and knee extension, crook-lying**. Lying on your back, with a pillow under your head, knees bent and arms alongside you, tighten your abdominal muscles to tilt your pelvis backwards slightly; lift your hips up; straighten one knee to lift the foot into the air, keeping your thighs level; bend the knee to put the foot down; repeat with the other leg; then slowly lower your hips. 5–10 times.

2. **Sit-ups with pelvic stability**. Lying on your back with your knees bent, feet on the ground but not fixed, and hands on your thighs, tighten your stomach and lift your head, shoulders and trunk to bring your hands just beyond your knees, keeping your abdominals pulled in; reverse the movement with control. 5–10 times.

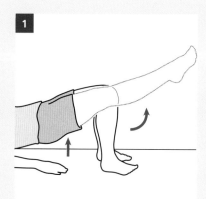

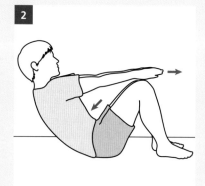

14

The Abdominal Muscles

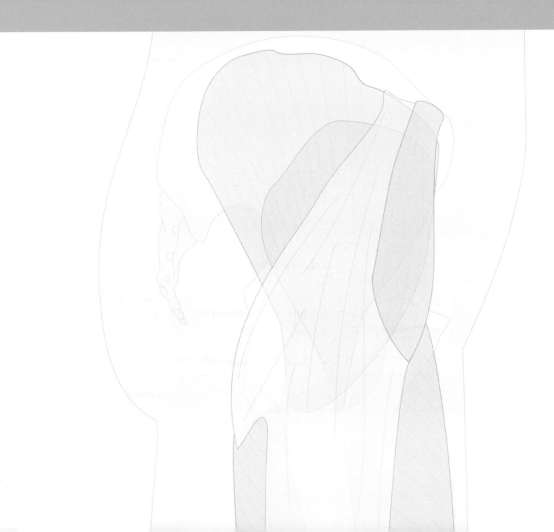

THE ABDOMINAL MUSCLES, SEEN FROM THE FRONT.

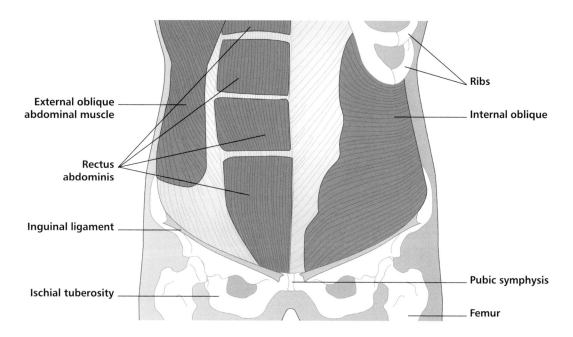

External oblique abdominal muscle

Rectus abdominis

Inguinal ligament

Ischial tuberosity

Ribs

Internal oblique

Pubic symphysis

Femur

The abdominal region is covered by four main muscles on either side of the midline: obliquus externus, obliquus internus, transversus abdominis and rectus abdominis. They link the top of the pelvis to the ribs.

Structure

The midline is a strong tendinous band called the linea alba, which stretches from the xiphoid process, the lower end of your sternum (breastbone), to the top of the pubic bone and the pubic symphysis. Just below the central point of the linea alba is your umbilicus, or navel (belly button).

Obliquus externus forms the outer layer from the side of the ribcage, linking the lower eight ribs to the iliac crest and the top of the pubic bone. In a slim, muscular person, when it contracts its fibres form diagonal grooves at the sides of the abdominal region, extending downwards and inwards towards the midline from the lower ribs. Obliquus internus lies under the external oblique, and links the iliac crest and pubis to the edges of the lowest three or four ribs. It also attaches to the inguinal ligament, joins transversus to form a tendon on the top inner edge of the pubic bone, and links into the linea alba.

Transversus lies under the other abdominal muscles, and spreads right round the abdominal region from the side of the body to the midline, extending from the inguinal ligament and iliac crest to the inner sides of the lower six ribs. In some people transversus is blended with the internal oblique, and some people do not have transversus.

The rectus abdominis covers the front of the abdominal region, extending from the pubic bone and symphysis pubis to the xiphoid process and the fifth, sixth and seventh rib cartilages. When it contracts, it forms horizontal ridges to either side of the vertical ridge of the linea alba.

What they do

Your abdominal muscles, especially the internal obliques, protect and cushion the abdominal organs and blood vessels, as there is no bony structure around the front of the abdominal area. The deeper abdominal muscles hold all the internal structures in balance, counteracting the effect of gravity when you are sitting or standing.

Efficient deep abdominal muscle activity is often referred to as core stability. It is the basis for good balance around the trunk and protection for the back. When the deep abdominals are activated, the abdomen is pulled inwards, making the whole area between the ribcage and the pelvis look hollow.

The abdominals work in all activities involving deep breathing, from yoga to sprinting. In the normal way, your abdominal muscles steady the chest wall as you breathe in, allowing the diaphragm to move downwards and create space in the lungs for the incoming air. If you tighten your abdominal muscles inwards as you take in a deep breath, your chest area opens up as your ribs press upwards and outwards. You create maximum space in your lungs when you create outward movement of your abdominal muscles as you expand your chest on the in-breath. When you breathe out forcefully, cough or sneeze, the abdominal muscles, especially the internal obliques, come into action.

During childbirth, passing urine or faeces, or vomiting, the abdominal muscles contract to exert pressure on the organs.

The abdominals come into action in all sports which involve trunk bending and twisting movements, such as racket games, football, kick boxing, throwing events and downhill skiing. In all trunk movements the deep muscles work in coordination with the superficial abdominals and the muscles of the hips, pelvis, ribs, chest and back. When you bend your trunk into flexion against gravity or a resistance, the abdominals, especially the recti, perform the action. If you lie on your back and lift your head a little way, you can feel the abdominal muscle activity with your hand. When you bend your trunk sideways against gravity or a resistance, the abdominals on that side contract. When you twist your trunk against gravity or a resistance, the internal oblique on the side you are turning towards acts, together with the external oblique on the opposite side.

The only time the abdominals are relatively inactive is when you sit or stand still.

Pain and complications

Unexpected pain or cramp in the abdominal region can be caused by a large variety of internal problems, including appendicitis, liver problems, urinary or circulatory conditions, stomach ache from digestive malfunction including irritable bowel syndrome (IBS), and gynaecological problems in females.

Stitch

A sudden unexpected pain in your side comes on during hard exercise.

What you feel
The pain is usually felt in the right side of your abdominal region, but can come on over the middle or the left side. It usually vanishes if you stop and do some gentle movements or stretching exercises. You may even be able to resume exercising after that.

Causes
Stitch is usually associated with energetic repetitive exercise, such as running, especially if you are not very fit, or have increased your training. Its exact cause is not known, but theories include spasm in the diaphragm (your main breathing muscle), gas in the large bowel, or contraction of the liver or spleen.

Directions
You probably need to improve your fitness through more gradual training. It can help to do breathing exercises (p. 204) and abdominal muscle stretching and strengthening. Eat and drink sensibly, both generally and in relation to exercising. If you eat a lot of fibre, you may need to cut down.

How long?
Stitch is usually temporary and transient.

Abdominal injuries

The abdominal muscles and their binding tissues can be damaged through trauma or overuse at any age. Injuries have a direct effect on the ribs, chest, lower back, pelvis and hips. They can also impair shoulder and leg function.

Hernia

Internal tissue, usually part of the bowel (intestine) protrudes through a weakness in the abdominal wall. If it happens in the umbilicus it is called an umbilical hernia. If close to the umbilicus it is a paraumbilical hernia. The tissue can become trapped, in a strangulated hernia. A hernia can happen at any age. The problem is most common in babies, but it can happen in adults, especially people who are overweight, or females during and after pregnancy.

What you feel
You notice a lump appearing in the abdominal region, which may come and go. In an umbilical hernia the umbilicus protrudes outwards. It may or may not cause pain in itself, but coughing or sneezing can hurt. It is usually tender if you press it. A strangulated hernia can cause severe pain and bowel obstruction.

Causes
There is weakness in the abdominal wall or round the umbilicus, which may be present from birth, or may be caused by the tissues being overstretched through obesity, pregnancy or injury. Increased pressure from hard exercise, heavy lifting or abdominal exercises such as double-leg raises lying on your back can push the internal tissue through the weak area.

Directions
A strangulated hernia has to be treated as an emergency. In adults surgery is essential if there is a danger of a strangulated hernia developing. In babies the problem usually resolves itself by about the age of four. However, if the hernia is causing problems, surgical repair will be recommended. You should avoid activities which cause an increase in abdominal pressure, and make sure that your diet is easily digested. After surgery, follow your specialist's instructions. Generally, you should avoid strenuous exercise and heavy lifting for six months or more, and then build up gradually to your normal exercise regime. Isometric abdominal exercises like the double-leg raise should be excluded altogether.

How long?
6–12 months.

Abdominal muscle injuries

The abdominal muscles can be torn, partly torn or strained through trauma or overuse at any age. Sometimes trauma damages internal organs as well as the muscles.

What you feel
There is sudden pain caused by an accident or gradual pain resulting from your exercises or activities. The pain may be severe or slight. It hurts when you contract or stretch the muscles, or if you press on the injured area, and sometimes also at rest. Coughing and sneezing cause pain. There may be localized swelling and bruising. The injured area may tend to cramp up at night if you turn over in your sleep. If internal organs are also damaged, you may feel other symptoms as well.

Causes
Traumatic tear or strain can happen if you are hit in the stomach, especially when the muscles are taut, or if you overstretch or overcontract the muscles suddenly. Overuse strains happen if you overwork the abdominals, often through doing too many repetitions of movements involving the muscles, especially sit-ups.

Directions
If there is a danger of internal organ damage, you must go to hospital or see your doctor as quickly as possible.

How long?
3 weeks to several months.

Rehabilitation and recovery

Acute phase

Following any operation in the abdominal region, you have to look after your circulation (p. 27), and your practitioner will tell you which movements you can do with your feet, legs and arms. You may be able to do the non-weight-bearing ankle exercises (p. 66), essential VMO exercises (p. 112) and possibly some of the advanced shoulder mobilizing exercises (p. 266). Breathing exercises (p. 204) are especially important.

Early phase

As soon as you can become active, your practitioner will set you appropriate exercises, which may be gentle basic stretching and strengthening exercises within pain limits, like the ones listed below. These may be combined with basic strengthening, stretching and mobilizing exercises for the calves (pp. 80–81), knees (pp. 112–114), front thighs (pp. 126–127), hamstrings (pp. 135–136), inner thighs (pp. 144–145), hips (pp. 160–163), pelvis (pp. 180–181), chest (pp. 206–208), back (pp. 230–234) and shoulders (pp. 256–260). If you have spent a long time on bed rest, you may need to do the exercises for correct walking (p. 34).

Recovery phase

When you have recovered basic flexibility and strength, you progress to the advanced abdominal stretching and strengthening exercises, which are usually combined with advanced exercises for the rest of the body. Alternative fitness training (p. 25) can start when you have full function in the abdominal muscles. You should regain full flexibility, strength and coordination in the abdominal muscles before progressing to the final recovery phase (p. 308).

Basic abdominal stretching exercises

1. **Abdominal stretch, lying.** Lying on your back with a pillow under the small of your back, straighten your legs fully and stretch your arms up above your head; breathe normally, hold for a count of 6, then relax. 5–10 times. To increase the stretch, raise the support under your back, or lie over a Swiss ball.

2. **Abdominal stretch, prone-lying.** Lying on your stomach with your arms close to your sides, elbows bent, and hands palms down on the bed; gently press on your forearms and elbows to lift your torso up as far as is comfortable, raising your head and keeping your hips in contact with the bed; hold for a count of 6, then relax. 5–10 times.

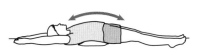

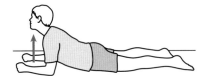

Basic abdominal strengthening exercises

1. **Abdominal activation, crook-lying.** Lying on your back with your knees bent, feet and arms on the floor, tuck your chin in and lift your head up and forwards, leading with your forehead and keeping your chin tucked in. 5–10 times.

2. **Abdominal activation, lying.** Repeat exercise 1 with your legs straight.

3. **Deep abdominal muscle control.** Lying on your back with your knees bent, one or two pillows under your head, tighten your abdominal muscles inwards, tilting your pelvis backwards just a little, so that your spine flattens into the floor; keep breathing normally; to make sure the abdominal muscles do not push outwards, you can check with your hands that they have tightened and created a hollow between the ribs and the pelvis. 5–10 times.

4. **Basic sit-ups (abdominal and trunk curl).** Lying on your back with your knees bent, hands resting on your thighs, and feet fixed or held down by a partner, lift your head, shoulders and trunk upwards to bring your hands up to just beyond your knees, keeping your chin tucked in; slowly reverse the movement and relax. 5–10 times.

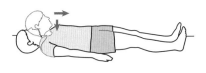

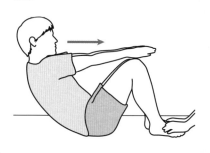

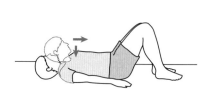

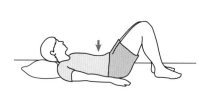

The Abdominal Muscles

Advanced abdominal stretching exercises

1. **Trunk stretch, prone-lying**. Lying on your stomach, with your hands palms down on the floor under your shoulders, lift your head and trunk up as far as you can, keeping your hips on the floor; hold for a count of 6, then relax. 5–10 times. *Variation: bend your knees as you lift your trunk.*

2. **Trunk and hip stretch, prone-lying**. Lying on your stomach, hold your ankles with your hands and gently raise your trunk and legs upwards to stretch the front of your body; hold for a count of 6, then relax. 5–10 times.

3. **Kneeling stretch**. Kneeling, lean backwards to put your hands on the floor behind you; arch your back to press your hips and trunk forwards; hold for a count of 6, then relax. 5–10 times.

4. **Twist stretch**. Kneeling, with a stick resting behind your neck and your hands at the ends of the stick, turn to one side, keeping your back arched and hips well forward; hold for a count of 6, then relax; repeat turning to the other side. 5–10 times.

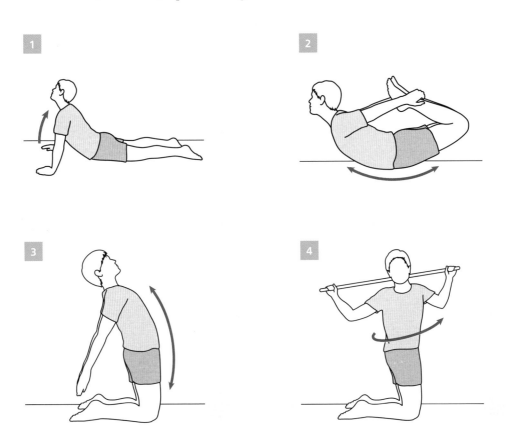

Advanced abdominal strengthening exercises

1. **Bent-knee sit-ups**. Lying on your back with your knees bent, feet free and hands resting on your thighs, tuck your chin in and lift your head, trunk and arms to reach just beyond your knees with your hands; reverse the movement with control. 10–15 times.

2. **Trunk flexion, lying**. Lying on your back with your legs straight, hands resting on your thighs, lift your head then your shoulders a little way, sliding your hands down your thighs; slowly reverse the movement. 10–20 times.

3. **Low abdominal and pelvic curl**. Lying on your back with your legs straight, bend your knees and bring them up towards your chest, curling your back as much as you can; reverse the movement with control. 10–20 times.

4. **Twist sit-ups**. Lying on your back with your knees bent, hands behind your head, sit up with a twist to take one elbow to the outer side of the opposite knee; reverse the movement with control; repeat to the other side. 10–15 times.

5. **Double-ended sit-ups**. Lying on your back with your legs straight, hands behind your head, bend your knees up towards your chest as you lift your head, arms and trunk forwards to touch your knees with your elbows; slowly reverse the movement. 10–15 times.

6. **Double-ended twist sit-ups**. Lying on your back with your legs straight, and hands behind your head, bend one knee up towards your chest as you lift your head, arms and trunk, twisting your trunk so that your bent knee touches the opposite elbow; reverse the movement with control; repeat to the other side. 10–15 times.

7. **Complex abdominal strengthener**. Lying on your back with your legs straight and your arms stretched up above your head holding a stick, bend one knee up towards your chest as you bring your arms over your head to draw the stick under your bent knee, then reverse the movement with control; repeat with the other leg. 10–15 times.

8. **Super abdominal strengthener**. Lying on your back with your legs straight and your arms stretched up above your head holding a stick, bend your knees up towards your chest as you bring your arms and the stick over your head; draw the stick under your feet and straighten your knees keeping your legs in the air, then reverse the movement with control. 10–15 times.

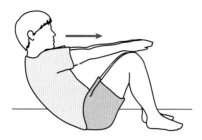

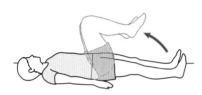
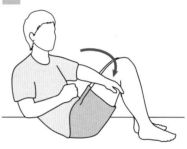
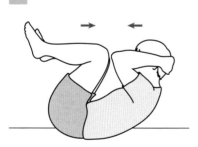
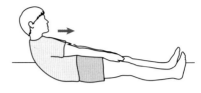
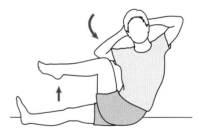

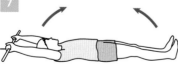
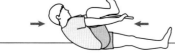
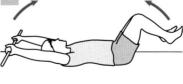

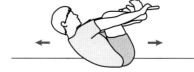

The Ribcage and Chest

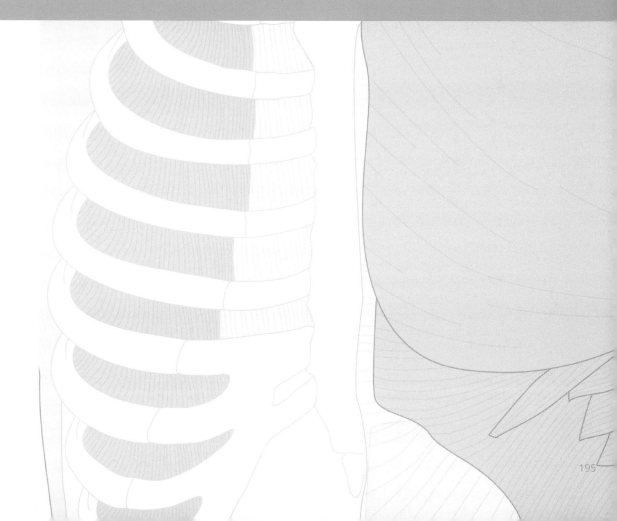

The Ribcage and Chest

MUSCLES AND BONES OF THE RIBCAGE AND CHEST, SEEN FROM THE FRONT.

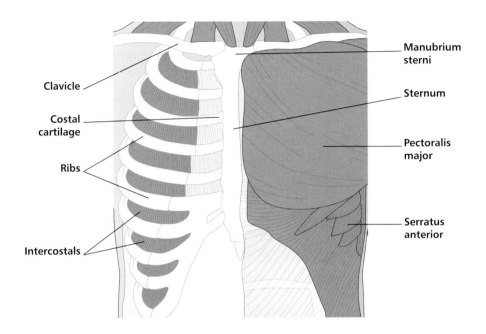

Clavicle

Costal cartilage

Ribs

Intercostals

Manubrium sterni

Sternum

Pectoralis major

Serratus anterior

The ribcage and chest form the upper area of your torso, between your neck and your abdominal region.

Structure

Bones and joints

There are normally twelve ribs on either side of the body, all linked to the thoracic vertebrae in your upper back. In your back the ends or heads of the ribs abut on the bodies of the vertebrae to form the costovertebral joints, which are classified as compound, complex joints. The ten upper ribs are also connected to the transverse processes (side-struts) of the vertebrae. All these joints have ligaments and capsules, and contain synovial fluid.

At their front ends, the rib bones join rods of cartilage at the costochondral junctions. The costal cartilages are like softened, slightly elastic extensions of the bones, although they feel hard if you press them with your hands just below the sternum (breastbone). The upper seven so-called 'true ribs' encircle your chest, and are fixed through the costal cartilages to your sternum on the front of your body, forming the sternocostal joints. Ligaments bind the joints. The second to seventh joints are surrounded by joint capsules and lubricated by synovial fluid, whereas the first is not.

The lower five are called 'false ribs'. Of these, three (or in some cases two) curve round forwards from the spine to join up to the costal cartilage structure, while the lowest two or three, known as 'floating ribs', are free at their front ends. Interchondral joints are formed where the sixth to ninth costal cartilages lie close together, and they are bound by ligaments and synovial-lined capsules.

Muscles

Deep-lying muscles

The ribs are linked to each other by the intercostal muscles. These connect each rib to the one below, and are arranged in three layers, external, internal and innermost, known technically as the intercostales externi, interni and intimi. The subcostals (subcostales) are deep-lying muscles in the lower part of the ribcage. They pass down from one rib to attach to the rib two or three below.

At the front of the body, transversus thoracis forms an internal covering over the chest, extending upwards from the lower part of the sternum to join on to the second to fifth ribs. At the back, the twelve levatores costarum are strong, short muscles which link each rib to the transverse process of the vertebra above it. Serratus posterior superior is situated in the upper part of the back, and links the second to fifth ribs with the vertebrae above. Serratus posterior inferior joins the lower four ribs to the lower two thoracic vertebrae and upper two or three lumbar vertebrae.

The diaphragm is a horizontal sheet of muscle which effectively divides your trunk into two. It is attached to the inner sides of the lower six costal cartilages and ribs, the front of the upper lumbar vertebrae and usually, but not always, the back of the xiphoid process, the lowest part of the sternum.

Superficial muscles

Four muscles cover the chest region on front of the thorax on either side of your body: pectoralis major, pectoralis minor, serratus anterior and subclavius. They link the front of your body to your arm.

Pectoralis major is the outermost and most visible. Its outer edge forms the fold at the front of your axilla (armpit), technically the anterior axillary fold. It spreads outwards from the sternum, clavicle (collarbone) and uppermost part of the external abdominal oblique, covering the front of the chest, to end in a tendon whose two parts are attached to the front of the upper end of your humerus (arm bone), just below your shoulder.

Pectoralis minor lies under pectoralis major, and spreads upwards from the front of the third to fifth, or second to fourth ribs near to where the bones meet the costal cartilages. It ends in a tendon which is mainly attached to the coracoid process at the top of the scapula (shoulder blade). The tendon may also attach to some shoulder ligaments and the humerus.

Serratus anterior is a large flat muscle which is formed in strips attached to the upper eight to ten ribs and the fasciae, or coverings, over their intervening muscles. It hugs the chest wall, passing round backwards to its attachment along the inner edge of the front of the scapula. Part of serratus anterior can be seen at the side of the body, roughly level with the upper part of the abdominals, when a muscular person does push-ups.

Subclavius is a small triangular muscle which usually links the first rib to the middle part of the clavicle, although it may extend to the top of the scapula.

Functions

The ribcage and chest muscles are active in all sports which involve trunk and shoulder movements, including boxing, the martial arts, gymnastics, racket sports, swimming, rowing, fencing and throwing events.

The ribs form a protective casing around your heart and lungs. The combined movements in the rib joints allow the ribcage to expand, rising and falling during breathing, especially when you breathe hard during strenuous exercise. The diaphragm is your main breathing muscle, and its action is also important for increasing internal pressure to help in sneezing, coughing, passing urine or stools, childbirth, or lifting heavy weights. The intercostal muscles help the action of breathing. They work together to hold the ribcage steady as the diaphragm moves downwards to allow air into the lungs. The external intercostals are especially active when you breathe in, and the internal intercostals when you breathe out. The two pectorals, major and minor, contract when you take a deep breath in.

Serratus posterior inferior pulls the lower ribs downwards, and the subcostals are thought to do the same. Transversus thoracis draws the costal cartilages of the second to fifth ribs downwards. The levatores costarum lift the ribs upwards, and serratus posterior superior may do the same.

Pectoralis major works when you pull your arm in from the side, or forwards from behind you against a resistance, and it also turns the arm inwards (medially) at the shoulder. It helps to draw your arm across your body towards the opposite side. It is active in lifting your body up and forwards if you do 'chins' to a bar or climb a rope, tree or rock.

Pectoralis minor works with other muscles around the scapula to turn the scapula downwards, holding it steady when you move your arm at the shoulder. Together with serratus anterior, pectoralis minor helps to draw the scapula round the chest when you reach forwards with your arm.

Serratus anterior helps to keep the scapula in place when you move your arm sideways or carry a weight in front of your body. It acts to curve the scapula upwards when you lift your arm above your head. Subclavius is thought to help steady the clavicle downwards when you move your arm.

Pain and complications

Heart, lung and certain internal abdominal problems can cause pain in the chest region, with symptoms that can mimic those of injury. Pleurisy (inflammation of the lining of the lung) can cause specific pain and spasm in the rib region. Some conditions such as shingles (herpes zoster) or injury in the thoracic spine can transmit pain or odd sensations round the line of the ribs through the intercostal nerves, which follow the lines of the bones.

Ribcage and chest injuries

Any part of the ribcage structure can be injured through trauma or overuse at any age. Injuries can cause difficulty or pain breathing. They can be linked to problems in the thoracic spine, neck, shoulder or abdominal region.

Traumatic fracture

The ribs and sternum can be broken or cracked in a traumatic injury. This can happen at any age, but is least common in children.

What you feel
The damaged bone hurts, especially if you press it. There may be a visible deformity if the bone protrudes outwards or is depressed inwards, with bleeding if the broken part pierces the skin. Sometimes there is obvious swelling. Bruising appears some time after the injury happens. Certain bending and twisting movements cause pain. Even normal breathing can be painful at first. Coughing and sneezing are usually excruciating.

Causes
Fracture can be caused by a direct blow, for instance from a hockey stick or a punch, or if you fall and hit your ribs on a hard surface. Ribs can also be damaged by a big rise in internal pressure in the chest, for instance if you are in a hunched position and take a deep breath as you try to lift or push a very heavy weight. They break more easily if you have mineral deficiency or bone problems such as osteoporosis.

Directions
If the injury is bad, especially if the sternum is pushed in, you need emergency treatment. You may need an operation. In all cases you should see your doctor or attend the casualty department to check that there is no damage to the internal organs, especially the lungs, major blood vessels or spleen. Fractured ribs and undisplaced fractures of the sternum are usually left to heal naturally, without immobilization or surgery, although in some cases taping might be used for comfort. You should gradually try to gain more movement in the affected area. If you feel you are going to cough or sneeze, you should hold your ribs firmly in place with your arms.

How long?
3–6 months.

Rib stress fracture

Any of the ribs can crack through overuse. This injury can happen at any age, but is least common in children.

What you feel
There is aching over the affected area, usually felt after exercise at first, but gradually increasing if you continue your sport. The pain eases if you rest for a few days, but returns with increasing severity if you resume the activity which caused it. If you keep trying to do your sport, the pain can develop to the stage where it hurts on simple twisting or bending movements, and when you cough, sneeze or breathe deeply.

Causes
A stress fracture is caused by repetitive muscle pull against a bone. The ribs can be damaged through intensive training for rowing, tennis or other racket sports, javelin throwing, weightlifting and baseball pitching. Bone damage happens more easily if you have mineral deficiency or any bone disease.

Directions
The stress fracture is usually diagnosed on the basis of the history of the pain and your activities. It rarely shows up on X-ray in the early stages, so a bone scan may be done if there is doubt about the diagnosis. You have to rest from any pain-causing activities, and do alternative training to stimulate healing. You must not try to return to sport before the bone has healed, as there is a risk that the fracture could become complete. You should allow two weeks after the bone has healed before restarting your sport very gradually.

How long?
6–12 weeks.

Costochondral injury

Costochondral injury usually affects one side only, but can happen in both sides simultaneously. Sometimes the costal cartilage becomes detached from the sternum or rib in a traumatic injury. More commonly the rib cartilages in the front of the chest become inflamed and painful. This is called costochondritis. The problem can result from a traumatic or overuse injury, but often the cause is not obvious. It can happen at any age, including in children. If there is swelling over the inflamed cartilage(s), the condition is called Tietze's syndrome.

What you feel
There is pain over the affected area at the front of the ribcage, which can be very severe or slight. You feel pain on movements involving the ribcage, including coughing, breathing deeply, twisting your upper body or stretching your trunk, so running hard, rowing, fencing, cross-country skiing or throwing the javelin can hurt, sometimes causing a clicking sound. It hurts if you press on the area. You may have pain at rest and in bed at night. In Tietze's syndrome you can feel the lump of swelling over the affected cartilage(s), and the skin may be red and warm to the touch. In costochondral separation you may see a visible deformity, which is either a protrusion or a sunken look.

Causes
Damage to the costal cartilages can be caused by overuse or faulty technique in sports which involve twisting the upper trunk, such as rowing, racket sports and throwing events. It can also result from being hit in the chest, perhaps by a fist or a ball, or from coughing hard over a long period.

Very often costochondritis comes on for no apparent reason, and is classified as 'idiopathic'. It can be linked to genetics, viral infection, or various illnesses and conditions, including ankylosing spondylitis (p. 170) and some forms of inflammatory arthritis or bowel disease. Some people have recurrent idiopathic costochondritis, although episodes can be months or even years apart.

Directions
Your doctor should check in case you have an underlying illness or heart disease. There is no specific treatment for costochondritis, so any treatment is usually aimed at the symptoms. You have to rest from any activities which cause pain, and avoid strenuous exercise and lifting heavy weights. If you have to cough or sneeze, press your hands over the painful area to counteract the pressure. As you recover, you should do exercises to help the ribcage move freely and fully.

How long?
2–3 months.

Ribcage and chest muscle injury

The muscles of the ribcage and chest can be strained or torn through trauma or overuse at any age. Muscle injury or spasm can happen together with injury to the rib bones, or as a reaction to underlying conditions such as pleurisy.

What you feel
There is mild or severe pain when the affected muscles are stretched or contracted as you bend or twist. There is usually tenderness if you press on the area. You may feel pulled down, with your shoulder drooping on the painful side. If the pain is severe, it can be painful to breathe deeply, cough or sneeze. Muscle injury, especially in the intercostals, can be as painful as a fractured rib.

Causes
A traumatic injury can be caused by a sudden excessive twisting movement, such as pulling against a very heavy weight, or trying to put the shot without preparation. Overuse can result from overdoing repetitive training, such as focussing on a single stroke in tennis or golf.

Directions
You should consult your doctor to make sure there is no internal damage or underlying problem apart from muscle injury. Avoid painful activities and start gentle movements to stretch the injured area within pain limits as soon as you can.

How long?
3 weeks to 3 months.

Intercostal neuralgia

The nerves which run between the ribs round the ribcage become irritated or compressed.

What you fccl
There is pain, possibly also tingling or odd sensations, in the pathway of the affected nerve(s). The pain travels in a band round the ribcage. There may be localized tenderness, and pain when you breathe deeply, cough or sneeze. Pain can be linked to movement, but is often intermittent and apparently arbitrary.

Causes
The condition can happen together with injury to the ribs, thoracic spine or intercostal muscles, or as part of an illness or inflammatory condition.

Directions
Treatment depends on the cause. It is generally aimed at relieving the symptoms, whether with injection, pain-relieving drugs, physiotherapy (physical therapy) or complementary treatments.

How long?
3 weeks to several months.

Rehabilitation and recovery

Acute phase

In all cases you must do breathing exercises within pain limits as soon as possible, to keep the ribcage elastic, according to your practitioner's instructions. Keep your neck and shoulders as relaxed as possible when you do the exercises. If you have an operation or have to spend time on bed rest, you must look after your circulation (p. 27), and your practitioner will recommend exercises such as the non-weight-bearing ankle exercises (p. 66), essential VMO exercises (p. 112), straight-leg raising (p. 115), basic hip exercises (p. 162) and shoulder exercises (pp. 258–260) as possible.

Early phase

You should progress to the advanced breathing exercises, and aim at making the ribcage movement on either side symmetrical. Chest stretching exercises should be started very gently, within pain limits, when your practitioner allows them. Strengthening work may start with isometric exercises, dynamic exercises or a combination of both, within pain limits. They should be combined with basic exercises for your pelvis (p. 181), abdominals (p. 191), back (p. 230) and shoulders (p. 258). Aim to do one to three sessions each day.

You should start alternative fitness training for the unaffected parts of your body as soon as possible (p. 25).

Recovery phase

As you regain strength and pliability in the ribcage and chest, you can add weight resistance to the dynamic exercises, starting with light weights and gradually building up. The exercises should be combined with advanced exercises for the related areas of the body. You should do chest stretching exercises before and after any other exercise session.

Before moving on to the final recovery phase, you should be able to lean backwards, sideways and forwards holding your arms above your head, and to twist to either side with your arms at right angles to your body, without pain or limitation.

Basic breathing exercises

1. **Breath control lying down**. Lying on your back with a pillow supporting your head and your knees bent or resting on a cushion, place your hands gently over the painful area; breathe out through your mouth consciously but without effort, taking care to empty your lungs completely; breathe in through your nose, taking a slightly deeper breath than normal; repeat 2–4 times, then breathe normally for 10–20 breaths. Repeat the sequence 3–10 times.

2. **Breath control, sitting**. Do exercise 1 sitting on a comfortable upright chair with your back supported, and your feet flat on the floor. If possible, your head should also be supported.

3. **Breath control, side-lying**. Do exercise 1 lying on your side with a pillow under your head, another supporting your upper arm, and another between your knees for comfort. Lie on the painless side first, then on the other, unless either is too painful.

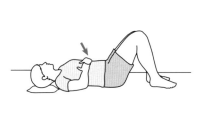

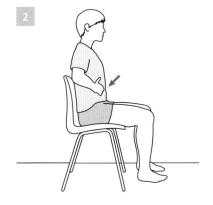

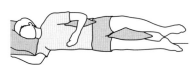

Advanced breathing exercises

1. **Deep breathing with rib expansion**. Sitting or lying down, place your hands over the lower ends of your ribcage; take a deep breath in for a count of 5, pulling your abdomen slightly inwards and letting your ribs swell up and out; breathe out for a count of 8, then relax completely and breathe normally for 10–20 breaths. Repeat the sequence 3–5 times.

2. **Deep breathing using the diaphragm and rib expansion, lying down**. Lying on your back with a pillow under your head and your knees bent or resting on a cushion, place your hands on the lower edges of your ribs on either side of the body; take a deep breath in through your nose for a count of 5, feeling your ribs and upper abdominal region expanding under your hands; then breathe out for a count of 8, letting your ribs sink downwards to expel the air completely; repeat 3 times, then relax completely and breathe normally for 10–20 breaths. Repeat the sequence 3–5 times.

3. **Deep breathing using the diaphragm and rib expansion, sitting**. Do advanced breathing exercise 2 sitting comfortably upright.

4. **Deep breathing using the diaphragm and rib expansion, side-lying**. Lying comfortably on one side, place your upper hand over the lower edges of the ribs on that side; take a deep breath in for a count of 5, feeling your ribs swelling upwards and your upper abdominal region outwards; breathe out for a count of 8, letting your ribs sink downwards and your abdomen inwards; repeat 3 times, then relax completely and breathe normally for 10–20 breaths. Repeat the sequence up to 9 times, doing two repetitions with your problem side uppermost for each one lying on that side.

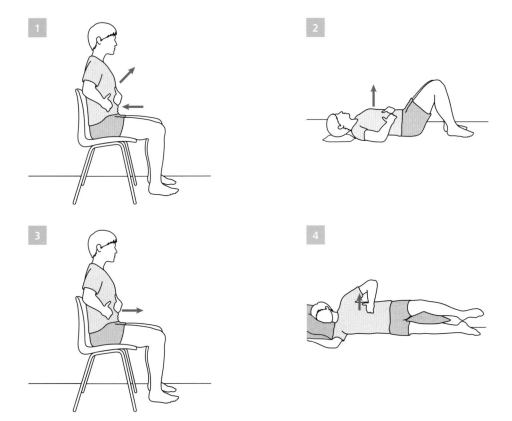

Chest stretching exercises

1. Sitting upright on a stool or bench, raise your arms sideways with your elbows straight and palms turned forwards; keeping your arms at right angles to your body, move them backwards as far as you can, take three deep breaths, then put your arms down and relax completely. 5–10 times.

2. Lying on your back at the edge on a bench or bed, take your arm out sideways, keeping your elbow straight and palm facing upwards; let your arm drop backwards towards the floor so that you feel a gentle stretch across the front of the shoulder and chest; hold the position and take three deep breaths, then bring your arm back and relax completely. 5–10 times.

3. Lying on your back over a Swiss ball or on a narrow bench, do exercise 2 with both arms simultaneously.

4. Lying on your back on a bench or bed with space above your head and a cushion under your upper trunk, hold a stick held in front of your body, with your arms shoulder-width apart and palms downwards; take your hands and the stick above and behind your head to feel the stretch across your chest; hold the position and take three deep breaths, then return your arms to the starting position and relax completely. 5–10 times.

5. Do exercise 4 with your hands held at different widths on the stick.

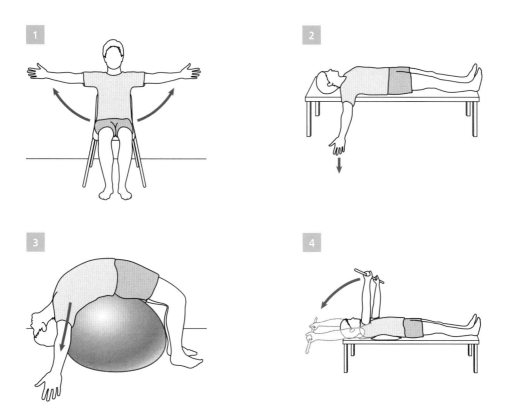

Chest isometric strengthening exercises

1. Sitting or standing with your arms held out in front of you, elbows bent and fingers pointing forwards, press the palms of your hands together for a count of 5, then relax completely. 3–6 times.

2. Repeat exercise 1 with your hands held up in front of your face, then held downwards level with your abdominal region.

3. Sitting, place your hands on your thighs with your fingers towards your knees; press your palms down against your thighs, turning your hands slightly inwards into pronation; hold for a count of 5, then relax completely. 3–6 times.

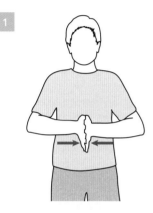

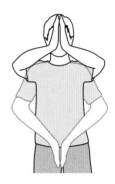

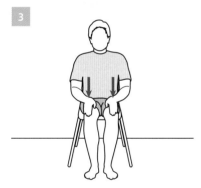

Chest dynamic strengthening exercises

1. Lying on your back on a bench, with your arms stretched out sideways over the side at right angles to your body, palms facing upwards, lift your arms vertically upwards to bring your hands together; control the reverse movement. 5–10 times.

2. Do exercise 1 with your palms facing downwards.

3. Lying on your back at the edge of a bench, let your arm drop downwards at the side of the bench, elbow straight and palm facing towards your body; bring your arm vertically upwards to lift it above your head; reverse the movement with control. 5–10 times.

4. Sitting on a chair or bench, with your arms straight out sideways and palms facing inwards, bring your arms forwards so that your hands meet, then reverse the movement. 5–10 times.

5. Use a seated chest press machine, or do bench press lifts. 5–10 times.

6. Use a 'pec deck' ('seated fly') machine. 5–10 times.

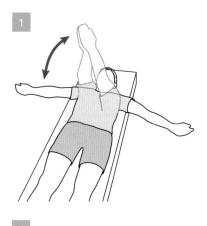

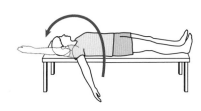

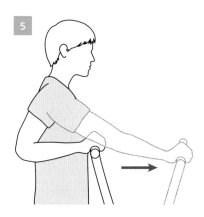

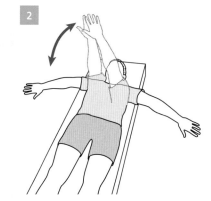

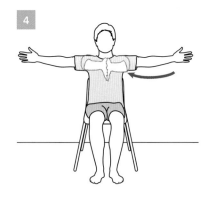

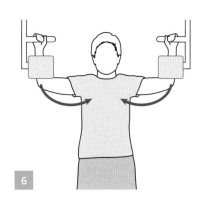

16

The Back and Neck

SUPERFICIAL MUSCLES OF THE TRUNK, SEEN FROM BEHIND.

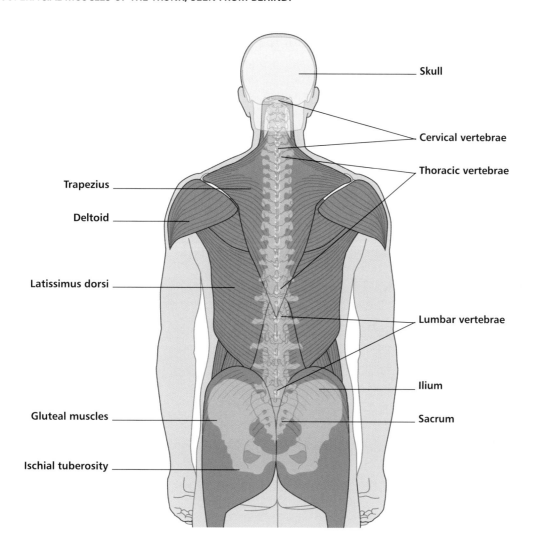

Skull

Cervical vertebrae

Thoracic vertebrae

Trapezius

Deltoid

Latissimus dorsi

Lumbar vertebrae

Ilium

Gluteal muscles

Sacrum

Ischial tuberosity

The spinal or vertebral column (backbone) extends from the base of the skull to the pelvis, forming three groups: the neck or *cervical spine*; the upper back or *thoracic spine*; and the lower back or *lumbar spine*. The top of the cervical spine supports the head; the cervical and thoracic spines link to the shoulder girdle and ribcage, while the lower end of the lumbar spine rests on the sacrum at the back of the pelvis.

Structure

Bones

The spinal bones are called vertebrae. Most people have five lumbar, twelve thoracic and seven cervical vertebrae, although the number can vary. The vertebrae are numbered from the top downwards, so the first cervical vertebra (C1) is at the top of the column, and the lowest lumbar vertebra (L5) at the bottom.

The majority of the vertebrae are cylindrical blocks of bone arranged one above the other, separated by shock-absorbing discs. The cylindrical blocks are called vertebral bodies, and they form the most solid part of the spinal structure. Behind the vertebral body is a roughly triangular arrangement of finer bones, called the vertebral arch, which forms a space called the vertebral foramen. Each arch has small struts protruding from either side, facing slightly upwards, downwards or backwards. They are arranged to form enclosed gaps between the bones called intervertebral foramina. The main bony struts are the transverse processes at the sides and the spinous processes which protrude from the back at the apex of the bony triangle. The spinous processes are the knobbly bones that can be seen and felt in the centre of the back, especially when you bend forwards.

Two vertebrae are different from the rest: the atlas, which supports the skull (cranium), and the axis directly under it. The atlas is formed as a ring, without a body or spinous process. The axis has a small body and a spinous process, but is unique in having a knob of bone at the front, called the dens, which locks into a recess in the atlas above.

BONES AND SOME MUSCLES OF THE NECK, SEEN FROM THE FRONT.

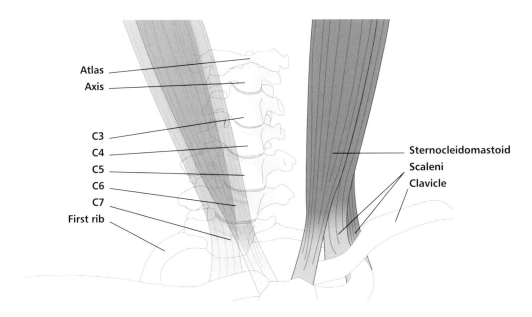

Discs

The vertebral bodies are simply arranged, one on top of the other, separated from each other by the intervertebral discs, except for the uppermost two, the atlas and axis. There is no disc between the head and the atlas either.

Each disc has a fluid-filled central part, the nucleus pulposus, surrounded by the annulus fibrosus, which is composed of fibrocartilage and collagen and forms a strong binding ring around the nucleus. The discs in the lower back are the thickest, while those in the neck are much finer. In both these areas the discs are thicker at the front. The thinnest discs are in the upper thoracic region.

The discs account for about one-fifth of the length of the spine in a healthy young adult.

Joints and ligaments

The joints between the vertebral bodies are formed between the bones and the intervertebral discs, which are attached to the bones by a layer of hyaline cartilage. Technically they are called symphyses, and do not have synovial sheaths or lubricating synovial fluid. The bones are bound together at the front by the anterior longitudinal ligament, which runs more or less vertically from the base of the skull to the front of the sacrum. The posterior longitudinal ligament binds the backs of the vertebral bodies from the second cervical vertebra downwards. There are no ligaments at the sides of the vertebral bodies.

The little joints formed between the ends of the bones extending out of the vertebral arches are commonly called facet joints, and their technical name is zygapophyseal joints. These are synovial, containing lubricating fluid, and bound loosely in capsules. They are often classified as plane joints, but in fact allow more movement than that implies, as the surfaces are usually ovoid rather than flat.

The struts of the bones are bound to each other by strong ligaments to form syndesmoses, joints which do not contain synovial fluid. The ligamenta flava are yellow-coloured bands which pass vertically downwards connecting each of the main struts which project backwards from the vertebrae. The supraspinous ligament connects the ends of all the spinous processes from the lowest of the cervical vertebrae (C7) down to the sacrum. In the neck the ligamentum nuchae binds the spinous processes together. The supraspinous ligament and ligamentum nuchae stand out in the middle of your spine between the bony points when you bend forwards. The transverse processes are bound together by the intertransverse ligaments, while adjoining spines are held by the interspinous ligaments.

The atlas is connected to the head through the two atlanto-occipital joints, which are held together by joint capsules and the atlanto-occipital membranes. The axis joins the atlas at three synovial joints: a central one where the dens of the axis is held in place by the transverse atlantal ligament, and two lateral atlanto-axial joints at the sides.

Muscles and tendons

The muscles controlling the neck and trunk are arranged in complicated layers over the front, back and sides of the body. Some of the muscles are extensive and long, others short and small. Some control the spinal joints only, while others connect the ribcage to the thoracic spine, and the thoracic spine and neck to the shoulder girdle (p. 244).

The front of the neck contains many small muscles over the throat. The most visible muscle crossing the front of the neck from the side is the sternocleidomastoid, which extends from the top of the manubrium sterni to the mastoid process in the skull, just behind the ear. Underneath sternocleidomastoid are the three scaleni muscles, anterior, medius and posterior, which link the upper two ribs to the transverse processes at the sides of the cervical vertebrae. Attached to the front of the vertebral bodies and transverse processes in the neck are three muscles: longus colli links the vertebrae between the atlas and the third thoracic; longus capitis lies between the skull and the third to sixth cervical vertebrae; and rectus capitis anterior joins the atlas to the skull.

The Back and Neck

DEEP MUSCLES OF THE TRUNK, SEEN FROM BEHIND.

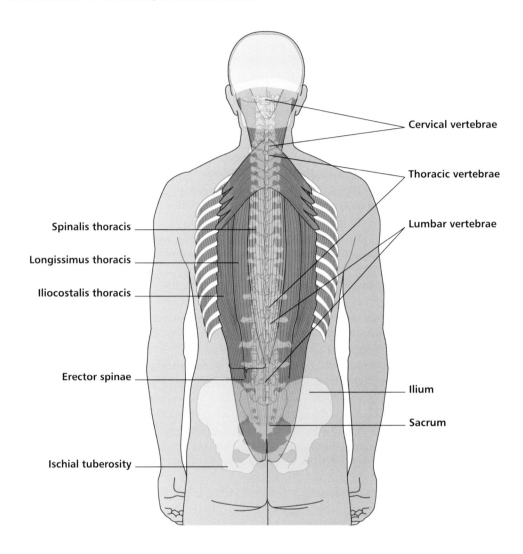

Cervical vertebrae

Thoracic vertebrae

Lumbar vertebrae

Spinalis thoracis

Longissimus thoracis

Iliocostalis thoracis

Erector spinae

Ilium

Sacrum

Ischial tuberosity

The back and side of the neck are covered on either side by trapezius (p. 211), under which are smaller muscles linking the cervical and thoracic vertebrae, while the suboccipital muscles connect the axis and atlas to the base of the skull.

Extending up the whole back in a vertical line from the sacrum to the neck are the back extensor muscles, technically called erector spinae or sacrospinalis, which are attached to the spinous and/or transverse processes at the back and side of each vertebra in its path. Erector spinae is formed in separate parts which lie close to the spine. You can feel and see the muscle group on either side of the lumbar spine where it lies under the skin, especially in a muscular person. Below the ribcage in the upper lumbar region erector spinae divides into three parts, with spinalis closest to the spine, longissimus next to spinalis and iliocostocervicalis forming the outer strand. Subdivisions as the muscles pass up the back give the muscles special names according to their shape and position. Iliocostocervicalis attaches to the ribs and the lumbar, thoracic and cervical spines, so it is iliocostalis lumborum in the lower back, iliocostalis thoracis in the upper back and iliocostalis cervicis in the neck. Longissimus and spinalis spread upwards from the upper back to the neck, then to the back of the head, as longissimus and spinalis thoracis, cervicis and capitis.

The transversospinalis muscle group is a complex grouping of small muscles which connect the spinous and transverse processes of the vertebrae. The interspinales link the spinous processes and the intertransversarii connect the transverse processes. Semispinalis, multifidus and the rotator muscles spread upwards and inwards to connect the transverse processes of the vertebrae to the spinous processes of the vertebrae above. Semispinalis and the rotators are subdivided into three sections, covering different parts of the spine: semispinalis thoracis is in the upper back; semispinalis cervicis links the thoracic spine to the neck; and semispinalis capitis extends from the thoracic spine to the back of the skull. The rotators are stronger in the thoracic spine than in the lumbar and thoracic spines.

Quadratus lumborum connects the top of the iliac crest over the pelvis to the twelfth rib and the transverse processes of the lumbar vertebrae L1 to L4. It lies under the back extensor muscles.

Spinal cord

The spinal cord, technically known as the medulla spinalis, connects to the brain through the medulla oblongata, and extends from the upper border of the atlas down to about the level of the first or second lumbar vertebrae. The cord is enclosed inside three layers called the spinal meninges: the innermost layer is the pia mater, the middle layer the arachnoid mater and the outermost is the dura mater. Cerebrospinal fluid flows in the subarachnoid space between the pia mater and arachnoid mater. The end point of the spinal cord is called the filum terminale, which goes down to the upper part of the back of the coccyx (tail bone).

The spinal cord lies behind the vertebrae, and is held within the vertebral foramina. Fine sensory and motor nerves run off sideways from the central cord through the intervertebral foramina, to supply all areas of the body with sensation and the ability to control movements. As the spinal cord is shorter than the vertebral column, the spinal nerves at the end are longer than the rest, and are known as the cauda equina ('horse's tail') because of the way they spread out.

The spinal cord and the brain make up the central nervous system, while the nerves which spread out from the cord form the peripheral nervous system.

How the spine works

The vertebral column supports your head and the central area of your body, and transmits forces through muscle action when you carry or lift a weight of any kind. It moves as a whole, with each segment contributing to overall movement patterns through its shape and structure. The vertebrae form curves, which reflect and affect the way the spine moves. You can bend your trunk forwards, backwards and sideways, and you can twist to turn from side to side. The vertebrae create a system of small levers generating pliability coupled with strength and power, so you can do complicated contortions in gymnastics and yoga, or create powerful dynamic movements for activities like tennis, baseball pitching, powerlifting or putting the shot. The spinal muscles lock the joints in position to protect the abdominal contents and create stability and strength for lifting heavy weights or doing handstands and headstands.

Lifting a weight of any kind places significant pressure on the vertebral column, especially the discs. The stress is greatly reduced if you lift correctly. The weight should be kept as close to your body as possible; you should bend your knees if the weight is on the floor, and use power from your leg muscles to bring it upwards; keep your back locked straight throughout; if the weight is particularly heavy, take a deep breath in and lift the weight as you breathe out. When carrying bags or cases, try to distribute the weight so that you can use a rucksack on your back, or use both hands or shoulders. Carry two kitbags, rather than one big one, and use wheels where possible.

Spinal curves, gravity and posture

Seen from the side, the neck and the lumbar spine bow inwards forming a lordosis, while the upper back curves outwards in a kyphosis. Seen from behind, the spinal bones should theoretically form a straight vertical line, but in practice they are often curved sideways with a slight twist: this is called a scoliosis.

The spinal curves develop throughout childhood as part of normal growth, influenced by genetic, metabolic and hormonal factors. In later life they may change through degenerative processes associated with aging, such as osteoporotic changes in the bones which can make the thoracic spine more kyphotic. Throughout your life, the curves are influenced by your activities and postural habits. One-sided sports such as tennis, fencing, baseball, cricket and javelin throwing can create a pronounced scoliosis. If your hip flexors become tight and shortened through excessive running or prolonged sitting, they can pull the lumbar vertebrae and pelvis forwards, increasing the lumbar lordosis. Sitting for long hours in front a computer screen at the wrong height can cause flattening of the cervical curve. Hunching while sitting can increase the thoracic kyphosis and flatten the lumbar curve, while sitting crookedly or with your legs crossed can create or increase a scoliosis.

When you are upright, the effect of gravity influences how your muscles work. Individuals vary, but in general the body's line of gravity passes down through the top of the head, between the ears, through the dens of the atlas, just in front of the second thoracic vertebra, through the centre of the body of the twelfth thoracic vertebra, through the back of the body of the fifth lumbar vertebra, just in front of the sacrum, slightly behind the hip joints, slightly to the front of the knee joints, and down to the ground between the feet, just in front of the level of the ankles. In the upright position there are always small muscular adjustments going on, mainly in the short muscles between the vertebrae, according to your posture and individual structure.

Poor posture can contribute to problems in the vertebral column. Good posture helps prevent injury and is a vital part of recovery from spinal problems.

Movements and muscles

The neck has its greatest freedom of movement forwards and backwards, so you can tuck your chin on to your chest or turn your head upwards to look at the sky. The atlanto-occipital joint allows mainly for forward bending, as in nodding your head. The atlanto-axial joint allows the head to swivel from side to side in a wide arc, as in shaking your head. Rotation is relatively limited in the rest of the cervical vertebrae. Side flexion of the neck is restricted, and generally involves some rotation.

The thoracic spine has very limited forward, backward and sideways movement, but greater freedom in rotation. By contrast, there is very little rotation in the lumbar spine, where bending backwards is the freest movement.

The muscles in front of the spine on either side work together on both sides to bend it forwards against gravity or a resistance: these are mainly longus cervicis, rectus capitis, sternocleidomastoid and the scaleni in the neck, and rectus abdominis (pp. 185–186) and the hip flexors (p. 149) lower down. When you are standing up, forward bending is controlled by the back and neck extensors, and the flexor muscles play little part in the movement apart from initiating it.

When you move the spine backwards against gravity or a resistance, the action is effected in the neck and upper back by rectus capitis posterior, obliquus capitis superior, the splenii, the semispinales and the upper part of trapezius, and lower down by the erector spinae complex and quadratus lumborum on either side. The abdominal muscles lengthen out eccentrically to control backward bending when you are upright.

The muscles on one side of the spine and abdomen create side bending (lateral flexion) towards the same side against gravity or a resistance. In the neck the active muscles are rectus capitis lateralis, semispinalis capitis, splenius capitis, sternocleidomastoid and the upper part of trapezius, with longissimus, iliocostocervicalis, the oblique abdominal muscles and quadratus lumborum acting on the trunk. When you are upright and bend to one side, the side-trunk muscles on the opposite side control the movement, while the muscles on the same side are only active at the very start.

The rotator muscles create the spine's twisting movements, mainly obliquus capitis superior, rectus capitis posterior minor, splenius capitis, sternocleidomastoid, splenius cervicis, the rotatores, multifidus and the oblique abdominals.

Pain and complications

The back and neck are prone to pain when the body's immune system is depressed or depleted. Dehydration is often a factor. Many conditions can cause back pain and related nerve symptoms, including ankylosing spondylitis (p. 170), inflammatory arthritis (p. 12), tuberculosis and tumours. Gynaecological and menstrual problems (p. 14) or disruption in the internal organs (p. 12) can be reflected into the back. Kidney stones can cause severe back pain and muscle spasm.

There are viruses which attack the spinal nerves directly. Illnesses such as glandular fever and meningitis are often accompanied by acute neck pain. Chest problems such as pleurisy can cause pain in the thoracic region. Common infections such as influenza can bring on neck or back pain (p. 13).

Back and neck injuries

Any of the structures in the back and neck can be injured through trauma or overuse. If you are dehydrated to any degree, the muscle spasm associated with injury is more intense. Muscle imbalance, weakness or tightness anywhere around the trunk, shoulders or hips can make you more vulnerable to overuse injuries. Spinal injuries can have a direct effect on the arms or legs, and range from debilitating to disabling. Back problems easily become chronic or recurrent if you do not rehabilitate fully, especially if you are careless about your everyday posture.

Referred pain

The spinal nerves can be compressed or damaged at any level where they pass close to the bones and joint structures of the vertebral column. This is often called a 'trapped nerve'. Injury can happen at any age, but is least common in children.

What you feel
You feel pain or a deep aching in the pathway of the affected nerve, often mixed with other symptoms such as tingling, hypersensitivity or numbness. There may be muscle weakness or a feeling of abnormal tightness. The symptoms can vary: you may have pain on certain movements, or with no obvious pattern. You may have no pain when you are active, but severe pain afterwards. Pain can be constant, making it difficult to find a comfortable position to rest in. You may or may not have pain in the spinal region where the nerve is compressed.

From the neck, pain is usually referred into the shoulder and arm, sometimes down to the hand. If the injury is high up in the neck it can cause pain up into the head and other symptoms such as numbness in the tongue. In the thoracic region the symptoms may travel round the ribcage. From the lower back, the pain travels down the front, sides or back of the leg, sometimes to the foot. When the sciatic nerve is affected, the symptoms are referred down the back of the leg, and this is called sciatica.

Causes
Compression of the spinal nerves can accompany any spinal injury, whether major or minor. In later middle age degenerative changes can cause narrowing of the spinal canal, a condition called spinal stenosis. Very rarely, stenosis is congenital and causes symptoms in early middle age.

Directions
A supportive corset or brace might help. Even if certain movements or activities seem to relieve your symptoms, be careful not to overdo them, as a severe backlash may follow. Your practitioner will try to identify the cause of the referred pain. Possible treatments include traction, manipulations and manual therapy, combined with special remedial exercise regimes. In some cases you may be offered injections or surgery.

How long?
6 weeks to a year or more.

Piriformis syndrome

The piriformis muscle becomes tight and presses on the sciatic nerve, which normally lies under the muscle, but in some cases passes through it. Occasionally there is also pressure on the pudendal nerve which controls the bowel and bladder muscles. This is usually an overuse syndrome associated with muscle imbalance, although it can occur as an acute injury. It is mainly an adult injury, and can happen from the late teens onwards.

What you feel

The main symptom is pain, sometimes with tingling or numbness, radiating from the lower back down the back of the leg. If the pudendal nerve is affected, you may feel symptoms in the groin, and you may even suffer from incontinence. Direct pressure over piriformis can re-create the referred symptoms you feel. In some cases pain and weakness are felt on turning the hip outwards and pressing the leg sideways into abduction against a resistance. In other cases walking with the foot turned outwards relieves the pain.

Causes

When the hip flexors and adductors are tight and overactive relative to the hip abductors, piriformis can go into spasm, becoming stiff and engorged. Sometimes laxity in the sacroiliac joints and overpronation in the foot are factors. The overuse syndrome is associated with sports involving repetitive hip flexion with limited abduction, such as long-distance running, racing cycling and rowing. Traumatic injury can result from a fall with the leg in an awkward position.

Directions

Once the diagnosis is certain, your practitioner will recommend exercises to stretch the piriformis, hip flexors and adductors, strengthen the gluteals and stabilize the lower back. Corrective foot orthotics may help. You may be offered an injection.

How long?

6 weeks to several months.

Traumatic fracture

The bones which make up the vertebral column can be broken or cracked through compression, distraction or shearing stresses. The vertebral bodies usually suffer crush fractures through compression, while the transverse or spinous processes can be broken through direct impact or being pulled apart forcibly. If the broken parts of the bones are not displaced, the fracture is stable. Unstable fractures often involve dislocation of the joints. Spinal fracture can involve damage to the spinal cord, peripheral nerves, lungs, kidneys, spleen and other internal organs. Fractures can happen at any age.

What you feel
There may be much or little pain where the fracture has occurred. If peripheral nerves are involved, there may be tingling or numbness radiating into your arm or leg along the nerve pathway. When the spinal cord is broken, you lose both feeling and movement below the level of damage. A major injury is likely to cause clinical shock.

Causes
There is usually a violent force. Falling and landing on your back, head or bottom causes direct impact on the bones. Violent shaking of the spine can disrupt the bones and joints, for instance in a car crash where the head is jolted in different directions. Landing awkwardly on your legs or shoulders from a jump and twisting the spine can cause fractures in the transverse or spinous processes. Sometimes the damage is attritional: for instance crush fractures in the vertebral bodies can result from doing a lot of parachute jumps over a long period. Fractures happen more easily if your bones are weakened by mineral deficiency or bone conditions such as osteoporosis.

Directions
Any major injury must be treated as an emergency: if possible you should not be moved until professional help arrives. In more minor injuries, if fracture is suspected, you should go to hospital as soon as possible. Your back or neck may be protected in a rigid or soft corset or brace, especially if the fracture is stable and you can move around normally. Otherwise you may be kept in bed for the first period of healing, sometimes on traction. In some cases surgery may be needed to stabilize the fracture.

How long?
Minor fracture: 3–6 months.
Major fracture: at least 18 months.

Spinal cord injury

In a bad accident, usually involving major damage to the spinal bones, the spinal cord can be severed or damaged. Injury is termed incomplete or complete according to the degree of impairment. Spinal cord injury in the neck affects the whole body, and is termed tetraplegia or quadriplegia. Damage in the thoracic and lumbar regions affects the legs, and is known as paraplegia. Injury can happen at any age, but is most common in young men between the ages of 16 and 30.

What you feel
When the accident happens, sensation and control of movement in the area below the point of damage are impaired or lost. Functional loss depends on the severity of the damage and the level at which the spinal cord has been injured or broken. If the injury is high up in the neck, your arms and legs feel numb and immobile, and you may be unable to breathe normally. Your heart rate, sweating, body temperature and pain control mechanisms may also be damaged. Injury in the thoracic region can result in loss of control of the abdominal muscles and legs. In the lumbar region your legs are affected, often together with bowel, bladder and sexual functions.

Causes
Spinal cord injury requires a high impact force which causes compression, shearing or pulling apart of the spinal bones. High-risk sports involve high speed, potentially violent body contact, extreme body movements, or the possibility of falling from a height. The spine is injured more easily if your bones are weakened by mineral deficiency or conditions such as osteoporosis.

Directions
Any injury involving the spinal cord must be treated as a major emergency, with professional help engaged as quickly as possible. You may need surgery to stabilize the damaged area; otherwise you will be put on bed rest, possibly on traction. Once spinal cord injury has been confirmed, and the initial phase of shock has passed, you will be taught how to manage everyday activities, including how to prevent skin sores, which are a risk because of the loss of mobility and feeling. You will probably need to use a wheelchair, at least at first.

Spinal cord injury is not necessarily permanent. Some people make a complete recovery, others regain a good degree of function. Even if the injury is diagnosed as complete, a level of recovery is possible, even years later. Treatment by specialist neurological physiotherapists can help you to progress, at least to some extent, at any stage. Keep positive and realistic – take each day as it comes.

How long?
This is a long-term problem.

Disc problems

The intervertebral discs can be damaged through trauma or overuse, usually involving compression or shearing forces. Injury is usually called disc prolapse or herniation. The term 'slipped disc' does not have a specific meaning. The annulus fibrosus can rupture, letting the nucleus pulposus protrude through the gap. Less commonly, the nucleus pulposus can suffer direct damage. Rupture can lead to pressure on the spinal nerve roots, or, more rarely, on the spinal cord. Nerve pressure causes referred pain and symptoms. If the sciatic nerve is affected, the injury is called sciatica.

Disc injury can happen at any level of the vertebral column, but is least common in the thoracic region. It can happen at any age, but is infrequent in young people below the age of about 20.

Discitis is acute inflammation in a disc which can happen at any age, including in very young children. It can be present together with an injury to the spinal structures.

What you feel
In an acute traumatic injury there is immediate severe pain. A disc injury caused by overuse can be present without causing any symptoms. There may or may not be back or neck pain. If there is, it is present on certain movements. You may experience weakness in the affected areas, or difficulty moving because of pain. There is usually muscle tightness or spasm around the injured area. It may be difficult to find a comfortable position for sitting or sleeping. Sometimes a position seems comfortable for a time, but when you get up the symptoms recur with ferocity. Coughing and sneezing can cause severe pain.

When there is pressure on the nerves, there is usually pain, often together with tingling or numbness, radiating down the pathway of the affected nerve on one side of the body.

Discitis causes acute severe pain and stiffness in the back or neck.

Causes
Disc herniation in the lower back can be caused through lifting weights incorrectly, or landing heavily from a jump. It can also happen through repeated stress on the spinal joints, or pressure from sitting still for long periods in poor posture. Older people can be more vulnerable because of degeneration of the soft tissues and disc substance.

Discitis can result from an infection in the chest or urinary system, or following surgery on the spine. It has also been known to follow certain injections in other joints, such as the knee.

Directions
For a disc injury, you have to avoid painful activities or sitting still for any length of time. It may help to wear a supportive brace or corset. In the acute phase, you may be advised to lie down, with a little walking at regular intervals. Possible treatments include traction or various kinds of manipulation. You may be offered injections or surgery, according to the severity of the situation. Exercises have to be strictly monitored: if you do too much, you may feel good at the time, but the pain comes back very quickly afterwards. To prevent recurrence, you should do protective exercises indefinitely.

Discitis may resolve on its own; otherwise it is usually treated with antibiotics and rest, although some movement is recommended to maintain the lubrication of the discs.

How long?
Disc damage: 6 weeks to several months.
Discitis: 6–12 weeks.

Stress fracture

The bones of the vertebral column can be cracked or broken through overuse.

What you feel
Pain over the affected area may be felt only after exercise or at night at first, but gradually gets worse. Rest eases the pain, but it recurs quickly if you go back to your sport too soon. If the problem develops, you have pain during other activities as well as sport. The crack can turn into a complete fracture, or lead to slippage of a vertebra (spondylolisthesis).

Causes
Overtraining in a sport involving repetitive movements is the most common cause. You may have changed your routine, increased your training or resumed your sport too quickly after time off. You are more likely to suffer a stress fracture if you have mineral deficiency or a bone condition such as osteoporosis.

Directions
You must avoid painful activities until the bone is fully healed. A supportive corset or brace can help. You should do painless exercises and alternative training to stimulate healing, according to your practitioner's instructions. Allow at least two weeks after the fracture has healed before restarting your sport in gradual stages.

How long?
3–6 months.

Spondylolysis

Part of the bony arch at the back of a vertebra is defective, or it can crack or break. This is usually a type of stress fracture and occurs as an overuse syndrome. It can happen at any level, but is most common in the lower back. It is especially common in teenagers and young adults.

What you feel
Spondylolysis does not necessarily cause symptoms, but if it does there may be pain on one side of the vertebral column, which is worse with activity and eased by rest. You may have pain when you cough or sneeze.

Causes
Sometimes the bones fail to fuse properly during growth, leaving a defect. Very often the problem is caused by repetitive movements which bend, straighten and twist the spine.

Directions
The defect is usually identified by an oblique-view X-ray, taken sideways on at an angle. You have to avoid painful activities, and may be advised to use a supportive brace or corset for the first phase of healing. Usually conservative treatment and remedial exercises are sufficient for cure, but, if not, you may be offered an operation to stabilize the bones.

How long?
3–12 months.

Spondylolisthesis

A vertebral body can slip out of place relative to the one below it. It can happen at any level in the vertebral column, but is most common in the lumbar spine. The slip is usually associated with defects or fractures in the bony arch behind the vertebra. It can be an acute traumatic injury, but more often comes on gradually through overuse. The problem can happen at any age, especially in teenagers and young adults, but is rare in young children.

What you feel
The slip does not necessarily cause pain or disability. You may feel generalized back or neck ache, sometimes with pain, tingling or numbness radiating down the nerve pathways in the legs or arms. If the slippage is in the lower back, you may have pain straightening your back, for instance when you stand up from sitting. Walking may be difficult. Coughing and sneezing tend to be painful. You may have pain on certain activities, which rest eases.

Causes
Spondylolisthesis can be congenital. As an overuse injury it can occur through excessive repetitive training involving bending and straightening the spine under load or pressure. In later middle age the problem can be linked to degeneration of the spinal structures. Traumatic spondylolisthesis can arise through a sudden hard knock or a bad fall.

Directions
The slippage is usually identified through an X-ray taken sideways on, although your practitioner or specialist may order other investigations if necessary. You may need a protective brace or collar, or even a plaster cast, to prevent harmful movements. Usually conservative treatment with rehabilitation exercises is sufficient, but if the slippage is unstable and causes severe symptoms, you may be offered an operation.

How long?
3–24 months.

Scheuermann's disease

The vertebrae develop unevenly due to osteochondrosis (disruption in the bone cartilage), resulting in exaggerated curvatures in the spinal column. The thoracic spine is most often affected, and the result can be a hunchback, or kyphosis. This is a growth problem which becomes apparent in the teenage years.

What you feel
There may be pain during sports, especially those involving twisting and turning. Sitting or standing still for long periods can also hurt. Trying to straighten your back is extremely painful and usually impossible.

Causes
The exact cause is unknown, and may involve many factors, including genetic.

Directions
Most often treatment consists of a specialized exercise programme. If the condition is severe and causing problems with the internal organs, you may be offered an operation.

How long?
The condition is self-limiting and stops when growth is complete, although any deformity will probably be permanent.

Scoliosis

The vertebral column becomes crooked, with abnormal sideways curves which make the spine look C- or S-shaped seen from behind. This can happen at any age, and often affects young girls as they approach puberty.

What you feel
You may have some pain on certain movements or when sitting or standing still. It becomes increasingly difficult to sit or stand up straight. Certain movements become limited, and when you bend forwards you tend to tip to one side.

Causes
In some cases scoliosis is congenital. When it comes on later and the exact cause is unknown, the condition is termed idiopathic scoliosis. Quite often the condition develops because of sitting habitually in a crooked position or playing one-sided sports which involve twisting the spine. More rarely, the condition follows a traumatic injury or is associated with neuromuscular disease.

Directions
You have to try to sit and stand as straight as possible at all times. Your practitioner will devise a specialized exercise programme to maintain and improve muscle balance and movements. You may be fitted with a customized brace to prevent further deformity, and monitored on a regular basis. If the scoliosis develops beyond a certain range (usually about 50 degrees magnitude) you may be offered an operation.

How long?
This is a long-term problem.

Facet joint injury

The soft tissues binding the facet joints can be torn or strained, and in some cases the joint suffers impingement or is dislocated. The muscles over the joint go into spasm and become tight. This is usually an acute injury, but it tends to recur. It is most common in the lower back, but can occur anywhere in the vertebral column up to the neck. Injury can happen at any age.

What you feel
There is sudden severe pain over the affected joint, which feels tender if it is pressed. You may find it difficult to straighten your back. Your spinal movements are limited by pain, and you may even feel lop-sided. Pain can radiate into the back of the thigh if the problem is in the lower back, and this is called pseudosciatica. From the cervical region, pain can be referred down the back of the arm or into the upper back.

You may find some temporary relief by lying on your back or side and curling up to bring your knees towards your chest. Sitting and standing for any length of time cause pain. Coughing and sneezing can hurt.

Causes

Very often the injury happens through the simple movement of bending forwards and turning slightly, for instance to brush your teeth in the morning. Dehydration is often a factor.

Directions

You can use warm pads or ice if they help soothe the pain and spasm. Sometimes a soft corset or collar helps. If the pain is very severe in the acute phase, avoid sitting. Lie down as much as possible. Make sure you are drinking enough water. As the symptoms of facet joint injury overlap with those of other spinal conditions, your doctor or specialist may order tests, and possibly inject the painful joint. Manipulation can ease the pain dramatically. After the acute phase, which usually lasts five to fourteen days, your practitioner will prescribe rehabilitation exercises.

How long?

6 weeks to 3 months.

Soft tissue injury

The ligaments, joint capsules, tendons and muscles along the vertebral column can be torn, partly torn or strained through trauma or overuse, with or without damage to other structures. Diagnosis is usually imprecise. Non-specific pain in the lower back is often called lumbago, or simply backache. In the neck a traumatic jolting or wrenching injury is usually termed whiplash. Injury can happen at any age.

What you feel

Pain varies from a slight ache or occasional sharp stabbing pain to crippling agony. It may be localized or spread over a wide area. It is either constant or present only on certain movements or when you are in particular positions. You may be able to relieve the pain by changing position or stretching in a certain way. Your movements may be free, or inhibited by pain. There is usually muscle spasm, a kind of tight cramping over the injured area. You may feel you are slightly twisted out of shape and cannot straighten up. If your neck is held twisted and bent, it is known as torticollis or 'wry neck'. You may also have referred symptoms radiating into your arms or legs.

Causes

Sudden acute injury occurs through wrenching, twisting, compressive or distracting forces, very often through lifting a load awkwardly or overstretching. Overuse injury is usually associated with overdoing repetitive movements, especially under load. Contributory factors include poor foot mechanics or muscle imbalance anywhere in the body. Muscle spasm can be caused, wholly or in part, by dehydration or a viral infection.

Directions

Make sure you are drinking enough water. A corset or brace may help relieve pain. Your practitioner has to exclude significant damage to other spinal structures. Soft tissue injury treatment is usually conservative. You may be advised to rest completely in the acute phase. Possible treatments include manipulations or other kinds of manual therapy, followed by a remedial exercise programme. Corrective foot orthotics may be relevant.

How long?

10 days to several months.

Osteoarthritis (osteoarthrosis)

The joints of the vertebral column can suffer degenerative changes. There may be loss of disc space, thinning of the bone cartilage surfaces, joint swelling and the formation of bony spurs or little protrusions at the edges of the bones. The changes usually happen in later middle age, but can occur earlier. The condition is often referred to as spondylosis.

What you feel

You may or may not have pain. If pain is present, it can be localized, spread over a wide area, or radiating into one or both arms or legs. There is usually increasing stiffness in the spine, so you find it difficult to bend and straighten or hold yourself erect. You may have pain at night, especially when you turn over. You may notice increased curvature, especially in the kyphosis of the thoracic spine, and you may lose height. Your muscles may weaken and become tighter.

Causes

Wear-and-tear degeneration of the body's tissues is part of the normal process of aging. Degeneration is more likely to happen if you have had injuries which affected your muscle balance and spinal function, or if you were involved in sports or other activities which placed heavy loads on your back. Osteoporosis can be a factor. The problem is usually worse if you are careless about your posture or have failed to keep generally fit.

Directions

You need to avoid painful activities, but keep yourself as mobile as possible. Spinal function can be reasonably good even if you have severe degeneration. You may be offered various treatments to help control pain and improve function. If you have episodes of acute pain, a supportive corset or brace can help.

How long?

This is a long-term problem.

Rehabilitation and recovery

Acute phase
For an acute injury or after surgery, you need to look after your circulation (p. 27), and do any exercises your practitioner recommends, especially, if possible, the essential exercises for vastus medialis obliquus (p. 112) and basic shoulder exercises (pp. 258–260). For severe back pain, it is usually best to lie down (p. 28) or walk around, avoiding sitting. Do not lie, sit or stand crookedly, even if it feels comfortable at the time.

Early phase
Your practitioner will tell you when you can start doing basic spinal exercises. You need to restore strength and stability in the trunk by combining exercises for the spinal extensors with basic abdominal (p. 191), pelvic (p. 181), hip (p. 162) and shoulder (p. 258) strengthening exercises. Once the spine is stable, you will probably be advised to do basic mobilizing and stretching exercises for the spine, abdominals (p. 190), pelvis (p. 180) and hip (pp. 160–161). You may also be able to do some of the hanging exercises, which help to decompress the spinal joints. Hydrotherapy workouts in a pool can be helpful and enjoyable, but you must take care, as too much exercise can provoke a painful reaction.

Tips: Sometimes hanging and letting the back relax eases low back ache; if not, you may find that working on bent-knee sit-ups (p. 193, exercise 1) reduces your pain. The sit-lift exercise (p. 312, exercise 4) can help ease pain in the thoracic spine and shoulder blade region.

Recovery phase
Alternative training (p. 25) starts as soon as you have reached a reasonable level of strength and mobility. In the recovery phase you progress to the advanced strengthening and mobilizing exercises for the spine, pelvis and all related areas. Add gradually increasing weights or resistance to the strengthening exercises when possible. You should also stretch your leg and arm muscles, paying particular attention to the hamstrings (p. 135) and front thigh (p. 126). Your practitioner will work on helping your body balance by setting you exercises for your weaker or tighter areas.

You must regain stability, strength, mobility and coordination in the trunk and the rest of the body before embarking on the final recovery phase (p. 308).

Basic back and neck strengthening exercises

1. **Extensor muscle activation**. Lying on your stomach, bend and straighten each knee in turn quickly. 10–20 times.

2. **Trunk and head extension**. Lying on your stomach with a pillow under your hips and your arms alongside your body, lift your head and shoulders a little way upwards and bring your shoulder blades together, keeping your hands palms down on the bed; slowly reverse the movement and relax. 5–10 times.

3. **Trunk and head extension through range**. Lying on your stomach over a dorsal-rise exercise machine or with your chest and head over the end of the bed, and your arms by your sides, let your head and chest bend downwards; lift your trunk upwards, just beyond the horizontal; slowly reverse the movement. 10–20 times.

4. **Isometric neck flexor strengthener**. Sitting or standing, place both hands over your forehead; press your forehead forwards, blocking any movement with your hands and keeping your neck and head straight; hold for a count of 5, then relax. 3–6 times.

5. **Isometric neck extensor strengthener**. Sitting or standing, place both hands on the back of your head; press your head back, blocking the movement with your hands and keeping your head and neck in line; hold for a count of 5, then relax. 3–6 times.

6. **Isometric neck side-flexor strengthener**. Sitting or standing, place one hand on the side of your head; press your head sideways, blocking the movement with your hand and keeping your head in line; hold for a count of 5, then relax. 3–6 times on each side.

7. **Trunk and hip extension with arm lift**. Lying on your stomach with a pillow under your hips and your arms stretched forwards alongside your head, lift one arm and the opposite leg a little way upwards; slowly reverse the movement; repeat with the opposite side. 5–10 times.

8. **Hip hitching**. Lying on your stomach with a pillow under your hips and your hands alongside your body, draw one side of your pelvis upwards towards your ribs, stretching the other side downwards, keeping your legs parallel; reverse the movement. 5–10 times.

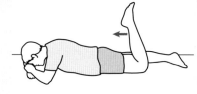

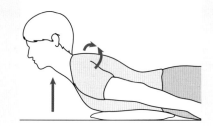

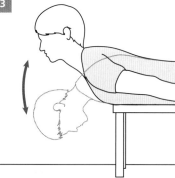

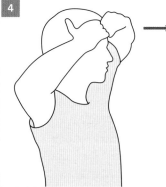

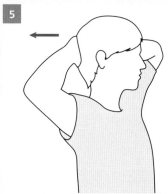

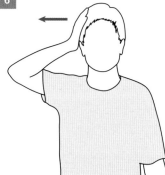

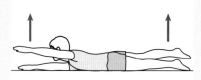

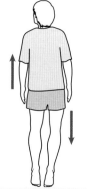

Spinal exercises in hanging

The bar should be high enough to allow your arms and trunk to stretch. If the bar is high enough for you to hang at full length, make sure you can step down from it, rather than jumping. If the bar is lower than your full height, bend your knees to lift your feet behind you to allow the arms and trunk room to stretch.

1. **Hanging stretch**. Hanging by your hands from a bar, let your trunk relax completely; step down when your hands are tired. 3–10 times.

2. **Hanging leg swing**. Hanging by your hands from a bar, keeping your legs together and your knees and trunk straight, swing your legs from side to side. 3–10 times.

3. **Hanging flexion and extension**. Hanging by your hands from a bar, bend your knees and bring them up towards your chest; straighten them downwards and take your legs behind you. 3–10 times.

4. **Hanging hip abduction**. Hanging by your hands from a bar, spread your legs outwards and inwards from the hips, keeping your knees straight. 3–10 times.

5. **Hanging hip hitch**. Hanging by your hands from a bar, draw one side of your pelvis upwards towards your ribs, keeping your legs parallel; as you reverse the movement, draw the other leg upwards. 3–10 times.

1

2

3

4

5

The Back and Neck

Basic back and neck mobilizing and stretching exercises

1. Standing with your feet shoulder-width apart, swing your hips round in a circular motion. 10–20 times clockwise, then repeat anti-clockwise.

2. Standing with your feet shoulder-width apart, arms straight out in front of you, swing your arms to one side, then the other, keeping them up at right angles to your body. 10–20 times.

3. Standing with your feet slightly apart, arms by your sides, bend your trunk sideways, bring the opposite arm up above your head, then reverse the movement; repeat to the other side. 10–20 times.

4. Sitting or standing, tuck your chin down on to your chest and turn your head from side to side, keeping your chin in contact with your chest. 5–10 times.

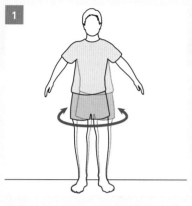

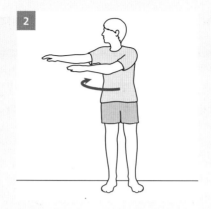

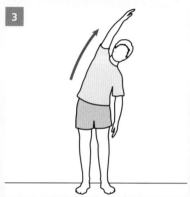

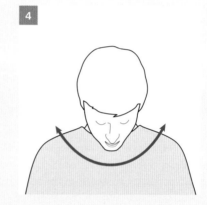

Advanced back and neck strengthening exercises

1. **Trunk extension with bent-arm raise**. Lying on your stomach, place your hands behind your head, elbows bent; lift your head, arms and trunk a little way upwards; hold for a count of 2, then reverse the movement with control. 10–15 times.

2. **Trunk extension with straight-arm raise**. Lying on your stomach, stretch your arms forwards alongside your head; lift your arms, head and trunk up a little way; hold for a count of 2, then reverse the movement with control. 10–15 times.

3. **Trunk extension with arm and alternate leg raise**. Lying on your stomach, place your hands behind your head, elbows bent; lift your head, arms, trunk and one leg up a little way, keeping the leg straight; reverse the movement, then repeat lifting the other leg. 10–15 times.

4. **Trunk extension with leg and arm raise**. Lying on your stomach with your arms stretched forwards alongside your head, lift your arms, head, trunk and both legs up a little way; reverse the movement with control. 10–15 times.

5. **Trunk extension with twist**. Lying on your stomach with your chest over the edge of the bed or bench, hands behind your head and elbows bent, lift your head, arms and trunk up a little way, turning to one side; reverse the movement, then lift again turning to the other side. 10–15 times.

6. **Advanced neck extension strengthener**. With a halter and light weight arranged safely over your head, lie on your stomach over the end of a bench or bed, so that your head and neck are unsupported; lift your head upwards a little way; hold for a count of 2, then slowly reverse the movement. 5–10 times.

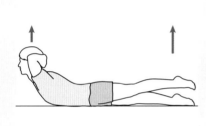

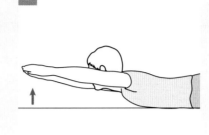

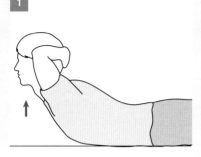

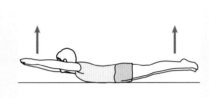

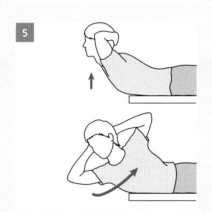

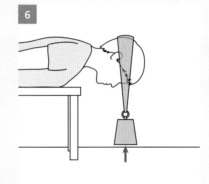

Advanced back and neck mobilizing and stretching exercises

1. Standing with your feet apart, bend forwards so that your trunk and legs are at right angles, and let your arms relax downwards; lifting one arm out sideways, turn your body to that side, letting the other arm swing across your body, then reverse the movement rhythmically. 10–20 times.

2. Standing with your feet apart, bend and straighten your trunk in gentle rhythmical movements. 10–20 times.

3. Sitting or standing, bend your head sideways and gently press it in the same direction with your hand; hold for a count of 6, then relax. 5–10 times on each side.

4. Lying on your back, place your arms out sideways or up above your head; keeping your knees bent, gently swing your legs upwards to bring your knees over your head; hold for a count of 6, then reverse the movement with control. 5–10 times.

5. Progression: repeat exercise 4 with your legs straight, and gradually work towards placing your feet on the surface beyond your head.

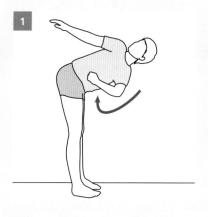

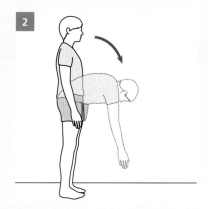

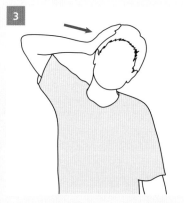

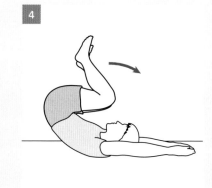

17

The Shoulder Region and Upper Arm

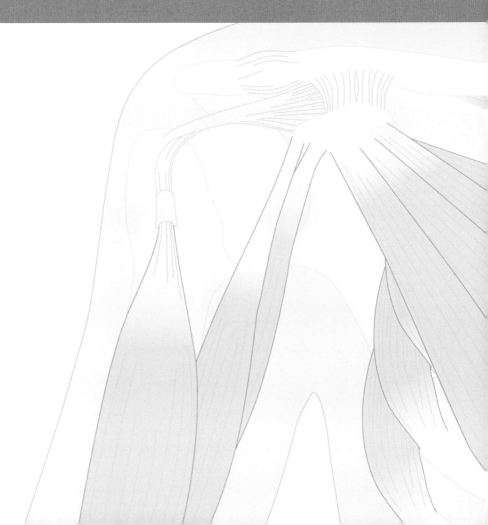

RIGHT SHOULDER, SEEN FROM THE FRONT.

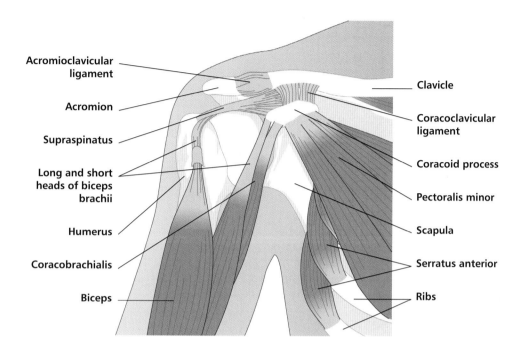

Acromioclavicular ligament

Acromion

Supraspinatus

Long and short heads of biceps brachii

Humerus

Coracobrachialis

Biceps

Clavicle

Coracoclavicular ligament

Coracoid process

Pectoralis minor

Scapula

Serratus anterior

Ribs

The humerus (arm bone) links the shoulder to the elbow. The arm is connected to the upper trunk through a linked complex of joints consisting of the glenohumeral (shoulder) joint and the shoulder girdle, which is also called the pectoral girdle.

Structure

The shoulder girdle consists of the scapula (shoulder blade), which lies over the back of the ribcage, and the clavicle (collarbone) at the top of the chest. The shoulder girdle is linked to the central part of the chest at the top of the sternum (breastbone). The shoulder joint links the humerus to the outer edge of the scapula.

Bones and joints

The shaft of the humerus is roughly straight and stick-like, with expansions at either end where it forms the shoulder and elbow joints.

The top or head of the humerus is rounded on the inner side, forming the ball of the shoulder joint, which is matched with a flattened area called the glenoid fossa on the outer side of the shoulder blade. The glenoid fossa is deepened into a socket shape by a fibrous rim called the glenoid labrum. The joint is very loosely formed, as the head of the humerus is bigger than the glenoid fossa. It is a ball-and-socket joint, technically classified as multiaxial spheroidal.

At the outer side of the top of the humerus is a knob called the greater tubercle or tuberosity, which you can feel if you press your fingers just below the point over the shoulder. Immediately below the rounded head of the humerus is a line called the anatomical neck, while the demarcation point where the top of the bone joins the narrower shaft is known as the surgical neck.

The scapula is flat and triangular, and lies over the second to seventh ribs. There are protrusions at the top of the bone which help form the links with the other bones in the shoulder region, and act as anchoring points for ligaments, tendons and other soft tissues. The coracoid process juts forwards from the outer part of the top of the scapula. Right across the back of the bone, in its upper part, there is a ridge called the spine, which you can feel with your fingers. The spine ends in a knob called the acromion, which forms the tip of your shoulder. Because the scapula moves across the back of the chest, it is considered a functional joint, technically known as the scapulothoracic joint.

The clavicle is shaped like a curved stick: it sits horizontally just above your chest, where you can see and feel its bow shape. The sternum is the central, vertical bone in the middle of your chest.

The acromioclavicular (AC) joint is the meeting point between the outer tip of the clavicle and the front edge of the acromion above the shoulder joint. It is classified as a plane joint. The sternoclavicular joint is the link between the inner tip of your clavicle, the breastbone and the first costal (rib) cartilage, and is technically a sellar (saddle) joint.

Capsule, ligaments and bursae

The shoulder joint has a capsule lined with a fluid-producing synovial membrane, which encloses the head of the humerus, and is attached to the glenoid fossa. The inner side of the capsule is attached to the edge of the shoulder blade, including the tip of the coracoid process. The outer side of the capsule is fixed round the anatomical neck of the humerus.

At the front of the shoulder, the capsule is reinforced by the three glenohumeral ligaments. The coracohumeral ligament links the outer part of the coracoid process with the humerus. The transverse humeral ligament lies at the front of the humerus and helps to hold the long head of biceps tendon in place. The least protected part of the shoulder is underneath, in your armpit (axilla).

Where soft tissues like ligaments and tendons cross over each other or lie close together, bursae (fluid-filled pouches) separate them to prevent friction. One of the biggest is the subacromial bursa, which lies between the deltoid muscle and the joint capsule, under the arch formed where the acromion and the clavicle meet.

Ligaments on the shoulder blade include the coracoacromial ligament, which binds the coracoid process to the acromion forming a little arch; the suprascapular ligament which bridges a dip in the bone just below the coracoid process; and the coracoclavicular ligament, which links the clavicle to the coracoid process.

The acromioclavicular joint usually has a disc separating the bones, at least partly. The joint is surrounded by a capsule whose upper part is thickened to form the acromioclavicular ligament. The sternoclavicular joint also has a disc separating its joint surfaces. It is surrounded by a capsule, and the bones are held together by ligaments.

Main muscles and tendons

Shoulder and arm

In the shoulder the supraspinatus tendon supports the joint from above, the long head of triceps from below. In front are the subscapularis tendon and the long head of biceps. Infraspinatus and teres minor lie behind the joint.

The deltoid muscle covers the whole shoulder, and consists of three parts: anterior (in front), middle and posterior (behind). It creates the joint's rounded contour. Its upper parts are attached to the outer edge of the collarbone in front, the upper surface of the acromion at the side, and the edge of the scapular spine at the back. The muscle fibres join up to form a tendon which attaches to the outer side of the humerus.

MUSCLES OF THE RIGHT UPPER ARM, SEEN FROM THE OUTER SIDE.

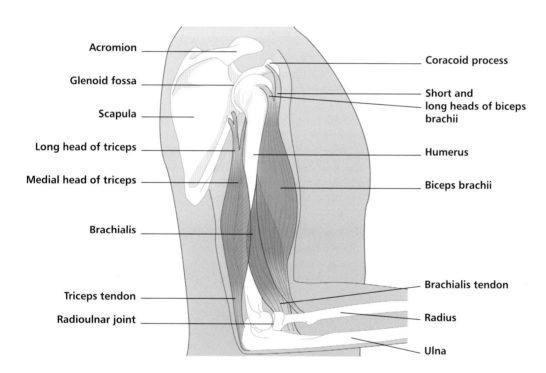

Biceps brachii is the most prominent muscle on the front of the upper arm. It has two heads: the long head starts as a tendon from a notch just above the glenoid cavity on the scapula and forms part of the shoulder joint, while the tendon of the short head is attached to the top of the coracoid process. The two parts come together to form the biceps muscle, which is the main bulky muscle on the front of the upper arm – the one that muscular sports players like to flex when they are 'pumped up'. At its lower end, biceps forms a tendon which is attached below the elbow, mainly to the back part of the radial tuberosity, a knob on the radius or outer forearm bone, although part of the tendon fans out to join the upper part of the forearm flexor muscles. You can feel the cord of the biceps tendon in the centre of the elbow when you bend your elbow and turn your forearm outwards, palm upwards, into supination.

Triceps is the three-headed fleshy muscle on the back of the upper arm. The long head starts as a tendon attached to a tubercle or knob just under the glenoid cavity on the scapula. The outer, lateral head is fixed by a tendon to the back of the shaft of the humerus, and is also attached to the lateral intermuscular septum, the band of tissue which forms a compartment separating muscles from each other. The inner, medial head covers most of the back of the humerus. The three heads come together in a tendon which fixes mainly on to the olecranon at the top of the ulna.

Coracobrachialis starts from the coracoid process, close to the short head of biceps, to which it is partly attached. It passes down beside biceps and brachialis to its lower attachment on the inner side of the humerus. Brachialis lies under biceps and extends down the front of the humerus to the upper part of the ulna.

Shoulder girdle and spine
The two rhomboid muscles, major and minor, lie over erector spinae (p. 214) and under trapezius (illustrated on p. 211). Rhomboid minor is attached to the ligament at the back of the seventh cervical and first thoracic vertebrae, and extends to the inner edge of the scapular spine. Rhomboid major lies lower down, and is attached to the spines of the second to fifth thoracic vertebrae, extending to the inner border of the scapula, below the edge of the scapular spine. Sometimes the two rhomboids overlap or merge.

Trapezius is a triangular muscle which covers the scapula. It lies over the rhomboids and part of latissimus dorsi, and is attached to the back of the occiput (skull), neck and all the thoracic vertebrae. The muscle fibres are directed towards the shoulder: those from the muscle's upper part fix on to the back of the outer part of the clavicle, the middle fibres go to the acromion and scapular spine, and the lower fibres to a tubercle on the outer edge of the scapular spine.

Latissimus dorsi, commonly known as 'lats' (illustrated on p. 211), is one of the body's largest muscles. It is attached to the spines of the lower six thoracic vertebrae, the ligaments down the spines of the lumbar and sacral vertebrae, three or four of the lowest ribs, and the top of the back of the iliac crest in the pelvis. It extends sideways and upwards, crossing the lower tip of the shoulder blade, to attach to the front of the humerus, in between the attachment points of teres major and pectoralis major. Latissimus dorsi and part of teres major, which lies under it, form the fold of flesh behind your armpit, technically known as the posterior axillary fold.

How the shoulder works

The shoulder girdle and shoulder joint work together whenever you move your upper arm. The combinations of movements available between the trunk, shoulder and shoulder girdle allow for complex skill activities like playing tennis and golf, throwing the discus, baseball pitching, cricket bowling, archery, basketball, handball, canoeing, and punching in boxing, tae kwon do or karate. Your shoulders can withstand strong compression and distraction forces. In gymnastics the joints are tested to the limit, for instance when you swing your body over the bar, hold the crucifix position between the rings, tumble, vault the horse or do handstands on apparatus or on the floor. Wheelchair athletes develop special strength in the upper trunk, chest and shoulders, depending on the level of the spinal damage.

Shoulder girdle movements

The shoulder blades glide around the ribcage. Movements in the acromioclavicular and sternoclavicular joints are slight, and occur only in conjunction with shoulder blade activity.

You can draw the outer edges of your shoulder blades upwards into elevation and downwards into depression, as in shrugging your shoulders. When you reach forwards or backwards with your arms, your shoulder blades glide forwards into protraction and backwards into retraction round the back of the chest. They glide upwards in lateral rotation, lifting the outer edges, when you raise your arms. They turn downwards in medial rotation when you press your hands down or clasp your hands behind your back with your elbows straight.

The scapula stays close to the chest wall as it moves, probably mainly through subclavius holding it in, while latissimus dorsi holds the lower tip of the bone in place.

Levator scapulae and the upper part of trapezius lift your shoulder against gravity or a resistance when you shrug it. Serratus anterior and pectoralis minor pull it downwards when effort is needed, and the same muscles draw the scapula forwards in protraction. Trapezius and the rhomboids draw your scapulae backwards in retraction. Lateral rotation of the shoulder blade is effected by the upper part of trapezius and the lower part of serratus anterior, while pectoralis minor, levator scapulae and the rhomboids bring the shoulder blade down into medial rotation when effort is needed.

Shoulder and arm movements

The glenohumeral (shoulder) joint is constructed to provide freedom of movement. Together the shoulder and shoulder girdle allow the arm to move forwards into flexion, backwards into extension, sideways into abduction, inwards into adduction, and up above the head into elevation, as well as twisting inwards into medial rotation and outwards into lateral rotation. Combining these movements to make circles with your arms is called circumduction.

The shoulder is loosely bound, so during normal movements certain muscles act to stabilize the head of the humerus. Subscapularis, supraspinatus, infraspinatus and teres minor are known collectively as the 'rotator cuff', and they stabilize the head of the humerus whenever the arm is lifted sideways. Supraspinatus counteracts the downward pressure of gravity, helping to hold your arm in place when it is down by your side. Biceps keeps the head of the humerus steady when deltoid contracts to lift the arm upwards. The long head of triceps supports the joint capsule, especially when you raise your arm.

When your arm is by your side, the anterior fibres of deltoid lift the arm forwards and up into flexion against gravity or a resistance, helped by pectoralis major, coracobrachialis and biceps. If your arm is behind you, pectoralis major initiates the action.

Deltoid's middle fibres lift the arm sideways against gravity or a resistance, with some help from supraspinatus, while coracobrachialis and the long head of biceps act to hold the humerus steady. Posterior deltoid combines with teres major to take the arm backwards, and with infraspinatus and teres minor to turn the arm outwards into lateral rotation.

When you hold your arm forwards and then forcibly pull it down and back against a resistance, latissimus dorsi and pectoralis major are involved in the first part of the movement until the arm is alongside your body, when the posterior fibres of deltoid and teres major come into action to take the arm backwards. Triceps helps this action, especially if you pull your arm in to your side, into adduction.

Pectoralis major and the anterior fibres of deltoid turn your arm inwards into medial rotation, together with latissimus dorsi and teres major. Subscapularis helps when your arm is by your side. Lateral rotation is effected by infraspinatus, deltoid's posterior fibres and teres minor.

Latissimus dorsi comes into action strongly when you pull a weight downwards from above your head, as in the lats pull-down exercise (p. 312), or when you use your arms to pull your body upwards and forwards, as in rock climbing or doing pull-ups to a bar ('chins', p. 312).

Pain and complications

Unexplained sudden or gradual pain in the shoulder region and shoulder girdle can be caused by inflammatory conditions or localized infection. It can be referred from other areas, including the heart, diaphragm, spleen, liver, gall bladder or stomach (p. 12). Unusual pain at the back of the shoulder girdle, near the shoulder blade, is often due to an infection or illness, including flu, glandular fever, pleurisy and chest infection (p. 13). Pain can be referred to the shoulder and down the arm from the neck (p. 219). Reflex sympathetic dystrophy (p. 10) is one of the causes of a condition known as 'shoulder-hand syndrome'.

Shoulder and upper arm injuries

The bones and soft tissues forming the shoulder and shoulder girdle can be injured through trauma or overuse at any age. Injury can disrupt normal patterns of movement in the arm down to the hand, also in the neck, chest, rib cage, upper back and pelvis.

Traumatic fracture

The humerus and the other bones in the shoulder can be broken through trauma which causes compression, distraction or shearing forces. Fracture can happen at any age.

The broken bone ends may separate, or stay close together. In young children the growth plates (epiphyses) of the bone can be disrupted. Soft tissues, blood vessels and nerves may also be damaged. The axillary circumflex nerve, which passes round the surgical neck of the humerus is especially vulnerable to damage when the upper part of the humerus is broken.

What you feel
There is pain over the injured area, bruising, swelling and possibly bleeding. Shoulder movements are difficult or impossible due to pain and/or muscle inhibition. Muscle wasting happens quickly. There may be visible deformity of the broken ends. If there is nerve disruption, you may have numbness or tingling spreading down the arm or up into the neck, and muscles supplied by the damaged nerve become weak and difficult to control.

Causes
Shoulder and arm fractures can be caused by a fall on to the shoulder, arm or hand, or a shearing or wrenching force. Bones are more likely to fracture if you suffer from mineral deficiency or weakening conditions such as osteoporosis.

Directions
Any major fracture has to be treated as an emergency. You may need surgery if the bones are unstable or if there is significant nerve damage. Otherwise the shoulder and arm are immobilized and supported in a sling. A traumatic fracture normally begins to heal immediately, and bone union usually takes about three to six weeks. The clavicle mends relatively quickly, whereas the humerus and scapula tend to take longer.

How long?
6–18 months.

Shoulder dislocation and subluxation

The humerus comes out of its socket, tearing the soft tissues which hold the joint together: if it stays out, it is a dislocation, whereas if it replaces itself quickly it is a subluxation. These traumatic injuries can happen at any age. The shoulder can dislocate in any direction, but most often the humerus moves forwards in an anterior dislocation. Dislocation or subluxation can happen together with fracture of any of the bones of the arm and around the shoulder.

What you feel
There is acute pain, your arm feels out of place, and you cannot move it normally. There is instant muscle inhibition, followed later by muscle wasting. There is a visible gap under the arch of the shoulder, compared to the other arm. There may be tingling or numbness round the shoulder, down the arm or even to the hand. If the humerus relocates itself quickly, the shoulder feels stable again, but usually remains painful on all movements.

Causes
In a traumatic dislocation or subluxation there is usually a violent wrench on the shoulder area when your arm is stretched out, as can happen in a fall while skiing or a violent rugby tackle. Muscle imbalance round the shoulder can play a key part: in butterfly swimmers, overdevelopment of the muscles on the front of the shoulder can lead to dislocation or subluxation of the humerus backwards through the weaker part of the joint, whereas backstroke swimmers can suffer anterior dislocation. Injury weakens the shoulder. Some people have genetic weakness in the shoulders, which makes them prone to apparently spontaneous dislocations. The more dislocations you suffer, the weaker your shoulder gets, to the point that it can come out through simple movements, such as turning over in bed at night.

Directions
Dislocation needs emergency treatment: the casualty doctor or surgeon may manipulate the arm back into place, sometimes under anaesthetic. The arm is usually immobilized in a harness or supported in a sling. If the joint is very unstable, you may be offered surgery. There may be a period of rehabilitation exercises beforehand so that you regain strength and mobility before the operation.

How long?
3–24 months.

Shoulder and arm stress fracture

The humerus and the other bones which make up the shoulder can be cracked through overuse. Stress fractures are more common in the humerus than in the clavicle or scapula. They can happen at any age, but are relatively rare in very young children.

What you feel
There is gradually increasing pain in the shoulder region, associated with sport or a repetitive activity. It may come on only after exercise or at night at first, but then becomes noticeable when you do your sport or any repetitive arm movements. The pain eases with a few days' rest, but recurs with more intensity if you resume your sport too soon. The affected bone feels tender if you press on it.

Causes
Shoulder stress fractures are associated with intensive repetitive activities which cause muscle or tendon pressure on the bone. There is always a change of routine: you may have built up your training schedule, practised a particular movement, style or stroke for extended periods on consecutive days, or resumed training after a lay-off. You may not have allowed sufficient rest and recovery periods within your training or competition schedule. You are more likely to suffer bone damage if your bones are weakened by mineral deficiency or disease.

Directions
You have to rest from painful activities for at least six weeks, or as long as it takes for the bone to heal. If not, there is a risk that the stress fracture will turn into a traumatic fracture and the bone will break completely. Meanwhile, you should do alternative exercise to stimulate the circulation, promote healing and maintain shoulder mobility. Unless the fracture has become complete, there is usually no need to immobilize the arm. After the bone has healed, you should allow two more weeks before gradually resuming your sport.

How long?
3–6 months.

Muscle and tendon injury

Any of the muscles or tendons at the shoulder and upper arm can be torn, partly torn or strained through trauma or overuse. Tendon strain is called tendinitis or tendonitis. Inflammation in the synovial sheath covering a tendon is called tenosynovitis. If calcium deposits form in a tendon, the problem is calcific tendinitis, which happens most often in the rotator cuff tendons.

Muscle or tendon injuries can happen at any age, but are most common in middle age or later.

What you feel

In a traumatic injury there is sudden pain over the shoulder. There may be swelling and bruising. In some cases there is deformity: if both heads of biceps rupture, the biceps muscle bunches up on the front of the arm. In an overuse injury pain usually comes on gradually and affects specific movements at first. If the injury becomes chronic, the pain becomes more general.

In all cases it can be painful to lie on the injured side, and there is wasting of the shoulder muscles, coupled with increasing weakness and joint stiffness.

When the rotator cuff tendons are injured, you cannot lift or twist your arm normally. Injury to the biceps tendons or anterior deltoid causes pain when you lift your arm forwards, or reach behind your back. Injury at the back of the shoulder causes pain when you contract the muscles to take the arm backwards, or stretch them by reaching forwards. Injury to the middle fibres of deltoid causes pain when you lift the arm out sideways, especially under load.

Causes

Trauma can be due to direct or indirect impact, or a shearing or wrenching force. Overuse injury is common in sports involving repetitive twisting movements against a load or at speed. The tendons are more vulnerable to injury if you have taken performance-enhancing drugs, especially steroids.

Directions

You have to avoid painful activities, and exercise the arm gently. Treatment is aimed at the symptoms. For a severe tear, or if there are complications such as calcific tendinitis, you may be offered an operation.

How long?

10 days to several months.

Bursitis

Any of the bursae around the shoulder, especially the subacromial bursa, can become inflamed, irritated or damaged through trauma or overuse. Bursitis can happen at any age, but is least common in young children, and most prevalent in late middle age.

What you feel
The area over the affected bursa becomes tender and swollen, and there is pain when the tendons and muscles around it are activated. In subacromial bursitis there is usually a 'painful arc' in the middle of the range: you can lift your arm sideways without pain to a certain point, then you go through pain for some degrees, after which the pain disappears and you can lift your arm up fully. It is usually painful to lie on your side. There may be pain at night, whether you lie still or move your arm.

Causes
Bursitis can follow a traumatic injury which has damaged other tissues. As an overuse injury it is caused by overtraining in activities like tennis serving, baseball pitching, cricket bowling, javelin throwing and water polo. It is more likely to happen if you have wear-and-tear degeneration (osteoarthritis) in the shoulder.

Directions
If the bursitis is severe enough, it may need surgery.

How long?
2 weeks to several months.

Impingement syndrome

Structures catch on each other and the shoulder loses its freedom of movement. Most often the greater tubercle impinges on the coracoacromial arch above it as you lift your arm. The rotator cuff and biceps tendons may be irritated or damaged. The problem is most common in middle age or later.

What you feel
The symptoms are similar to those of bursitis.

Causes
Impingement often follows other injuries around the shoulder, or is part of generalized wear and tear.

Directions
Surgery may be needed.

How long?
Usually several months.

'Frozen shoulder'

The shoulder becomes very stiff and the joint capsule tightens, to the point where it is almost impossible to move the arm away from the body. This problem, whose technical name is adhesive capsulitis, affects middle-aged and older adults, especially women. It can happen in both shoulders simultaneously, one shoulder after the other, or one shoulder alone.

Traditionally the term was used only for shoulder stiffness which came on for no obvious cause, but now it also covers immobility following an injury or surgery.

What you feel
You may feel constant pain, or pain on certain movements, together with increasing stiffness. In some cases there is no pain, just the feeling that movement is blocked. It hurts if you try to move the arm passively using your other hand. The muscles weaken and waste, so the bones of the shoulder look more prominent. Lying on the affected side is usually painful, and lying on the other side can also hurt.

Causes
The true 'frozen shoulder' comes on apparently spontaneously. It has been linked to various conditions, including thyroid dysfunction, diabetes and heart problems. In females it is relatively common around the time of the menopause, and it is possible that taking hormone replacement therapy has an influence. The problem is often worse if it happens in the non-dominant shoulder, because you use it less in normal activities and so do not counteract the stiffness.

Following a shoulder injury or operation, extreme stiffness is more likely to happen if the shoulder has been immobilized for a lengthy period, or if you failed to do the necessary exercises to recover full strength and mobility.

Directions
'Spontaneous frozen shoulder' usually eases by itself, very gradually. Any underlying factors or medical conditions have to be resolved. In all cases treatment is aimed at the symptoms, and usually includes massage and gentle mobilization techniques for the shoulder girdle, especially around the shoulder blade. More invasive techniques include injection, manipulation under anaesthetic, and surgery. Gentle progressive exercises are essential in every case.

How long?
10 days to 2 years.

Acromioclavicular injury

The ligaments of the acromioclavicular (AC) joint can be torn, partly torn or strained in a traumatic injury, causing instability, subluxation or dislocation. AC injury, which is also known as shoulder separation, can accompany injury to the shoulder joint and/or the sternoclavicular joint.

What you feel
There is pain directly over the top of the front of the shoulder, and tenderness if you press on the joint. It is painful to lift your arm right up above your head. If you bring your arms inwards tightly across your chest, you may feel and see the bones lifting upwards abnormally.

Causes
The most common cause is a direct blow close to the joint. You might be hit by a stick in lacrosse, suffer a violent shoulder tackle in rugby, or fall directly on to the point of the shoulder. The AC joint can also be injured if you fall heavily on to your hand.

Directions
The arm is usually rested in a sling for the initial healing phase. Depending on the severity of the injury, you may be offered an injection or operation. Progressive rehabilitation exercises are essential in all cases.

How long?
4 weeks to several months.

Sternoclavicular injury

The sternoclavicular joint can be disrupted or dislocated through trauma. The ligaments can be strained or torn, and the clavicle can be forced outwards or inwards. It is a relatively rare injury which usually happens in adults in conjunction with shoulder or AC joint injury. In the under-25s, injury pain at the inner end of the collarbone is more likely to be damage to the growth plate than sternoclavicular joint disruption, although the symptoms might seem similar.

What you feel
Pain and tenderness occur over the inner end of the collarbone, and the bone may jut out or sag inwards. It may also be painful to breathe and swallow.

Causes
A direct blow to the shoulder or chest disrupts the joint, or it is damaged in conjunction with injury to the upper chest.

Directions
The arm is usually rested in a sling for the initial healing phase. Sometimes the joint is gently manipulated back into place. In a severe or complicated case, surgery may be offered. In all cases, progressive exercises are essential.

How long?
4 weeks to several months.

Winged scapula

Nerve damage causes the shoulder blade to jut outwards instead of staying close to the ribcage when you move your arm forwards against pressure. Most often it is the long thoracic nerve controlling the serratus anterior muscle which is affected, but sometimes scapula winging is caused by damage to the accessory nerve which supplies the trapezius muscle, or to the dorsal scapular nerve which controls the rhomboids. Nerve damage can follow a traumatic injury in the neck or shoulder region, or can be due to an overuse syndrome. It can happen at any age.

What you feel
There is usually pain over the scapula and sometimes down the arm. If you try to do movements such as press-ups, there is weakness, possibly pain, and the shoulder blade sticks out.

Causes
You may have been hit over the area between your neck and shoulder in a traumatic accident. Overuse damage can happen through sports involving repetitive forceful arm movements. Nerve damage happens more easily if you have been ill with flu, tonsillitis or bronchitis, have suffered allergic reactions to drugs or have been exposed to pesticides.

Directions
If the problem becomes long-standing, you may be offered an operation.

How long?
3–24 months.

Suprascapular neuropathy

Damage to the suprascapular nerve causes shoulder pain and muscle weakness, specifically in supraspinatus and infraspinatus. This can happen in a traumatic accident which causes other damage around the shoulder, or as an overuse syndrome.

What you feel
There is pain or aching over the back of the shoulder and inside the joint. You may feel pain or tingling down your arm. You have difficulty lifting your arm out sideways and twisting it outwards. The muscles waste, leaving the shoulder looking slightly hollow.

Causes
Apart from a traumatic shoulder injury, damage is often associated with repetitive forceful overhead movements.

Directions
The shoulder is usually protected in a sling for the primary healing phase. If the problem does not resolve, you may be offered an injection or operation. Progressive remedial exercises are essential in all cases.

How long?
3 weeks to several months.

Osteoarthritis (osteoarthrosis)

Wear-and-tear degeneration can happen in any of the joints which make up the shoulder and shoulder girdle, and is especially common in the acromioclavicular and glenohumeral joints. The articular cartilage which forms the joint surfaces becomes roughened or pitted, and wears away; small bony outcrops called osteophytes can form at the edges of the affected joint; the joint capsule can become thickened; and fluid can gather in the joint, making it swollen. It is a problem which normally affects adults from late middle age onwards, although it can happen earlier.

What you feel
You feel pain on certain movements, and in bed at night. Your shoulder may feel stiff, giving a feeling of 'catching' or a creaking sound on movement. Aching may get better or worse according to changes in the weather. The muscles round the shoulder become increasingly weak and inflexible. If the problem progresses, the shoulder becomes more and more immobile, and you may find it difficult, if not impossible, to do simple actions like combing your hair or reaching behind you to put your coat on.

Causes
Joint degeneration is often a late after-effect of injury, coming on after several years. It is more likely to happen if you failed to recover full movement and strength following the initial injury, however trivial it might have been. Some people have a hereditary tendency to osteoarthritis.

Directions
Maintaining and improving joint movement and muscle strength are the primary aims of treatment, alongside reducing pain. The more you can maintain function in the shoulder, the less it hurts, no matter how bad the arthritis might seem on X-rays. However, if function becomes severely limited, surgery may be needed.

How long?
This is a long-term problem.

Rehabilitation and recovery

Acute phase

If you have surgery, you must look after your circulation (p. 27), and do general exercises as recommended by your practitioner. Exercises may include non-weight-bearing ankle exercises (p. 66), straight-leg raising (p. 115), essential vastus medialis obliquus exercises (p. 112), knee mobilizing exercises (pp. 113–114), and basic exercises for the front thigh (pp. 126–127), hamstrings (pp. 135–136), inner thigh (pp. 144–145), hips (pp. 160–162), pelvis (pp. 180–181) and abdominals (pp. 190–191). You should also work on elbow (p. 286), wrist and hand (p. 302) movements as possible. Aim to do one to three sessions a day.

Early phase

After any injury, especially if the arm has been immobilized in a sling or cast, the muscles around the shoulder will be weak. As the shoulder depends on its muscles and tendons for stability as well as for movement, the priority is to strengthen them, and to restore the right movement patterns around the shoulder, avoiding compensation through the trapezius muscle in the neck or the shoulder girdle muscles behind the shoulder. It is helpful to use a mirror, at least at first, to make sure you are doing all your exercises accurately. You may start with basic isometric exercises followed by dynamic strengthening, stretching and mobilizing exercises, all within pain limits. Your practitioner may use electrical muscle stimulation (p. 20) to help restore efficient neuromuscular coordination. Alternative training for the rest of your body should start as soon as possible (p. 25).

Recovery phase

Once the shoulder is stable and mobile, you can progress to advanced exercises. They should be combined with advanced exercises for your front thigh (p. 128), hamstrings (p. 137), inner thigh (p. 146), hips (pp. 164–166), pelvis (pp. 182–183), abdominals (pp. 192–193), chest (pp. 206–208), back (pp. 236–238), elbow and forearm (pp. 304–306), and wrist and hand (pp. 304–307), as possible. As the advanced shoulder strengthening movements become easier, you can gradually add weights or resistance for some of the exercises, where appropriate.

You must regain stability, strength and full movement in the shoulder and its muscles before progressing to the final recovery phase (p. 308).

Basic shoulder and upper arm isometric strengthening exercises

1. Sitting or standing with your arm straight by your side, place your other hand on the arm just above the outside of the elbow to block any movement; contract the muscles of the straight arm as if to lift it sideways, while holding it still with the other arm; hold the contraction for a count of 5, then relax completely. 3–6 times.

2. Sitting or standing with your arm straight by your side, place the other hand on the front of your arm, just above the elbow; blocking any movement with your hand, contract the muscles on your straight arm as if to take the arm forwards; hold for a count of 5, then relax. 3–6 times.

3. Sitting or standing with your arm straight down by your side, place the other hand over the back of the arm, just above the elbow; gently press your straight arm backwards, blocking movement with your other hand; hold for a count of 5, then relax. 3–6 times.

4. Sitting or standing with your elbow bent to a right angle and your palm facing inwards, place the palm against a fixed object; keeping your elbow by your side, press your palm against the object for a count of 5, then relax. 3–6 times. *Variations: keeping your elbow by your side, take your hand outwards at varying angles and repeat the isometric press.*

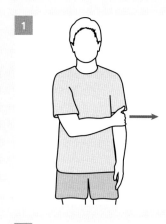

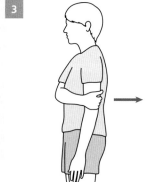

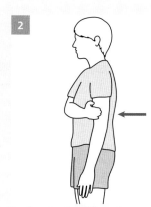

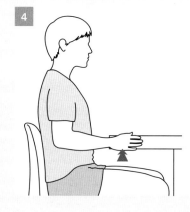

Basic shoulder and upper arm dynamic strengthening exercises

1. **Shoulder girdle strengthener**. Lying on your stomach, lift your head and shoulders a little way, keeping your gluteal (seat) muscles relaxed; bring your shoulder blades gently together; hold for a count of 2, then slowly reverse the movement and relax. 5–10 times.

2. **Arm abduction with elbows bent**. Sitting or standing with your back straight, head up and arms by your sides, bend your elbows to a right angle; keeping your elbows bent and neck relaxed, lift your arms up sideways to horizontal (elbows level with shoulders), then slowly reverse the movement and relax. 10–20 times.

3. **Arm abduction with elbows straight**. Sitting or standing with your back straight, head up and arms by your sides, lift your arms up sideways, then slowly reverse the movement and relax. Your palms can face upwards, downwards and forwards in turn. 5–10 times.

4. **Forward lift**. Sitting or standing, with your arms by your sides, elbows straight and palms facing inwards, lift your arms forwards and straight upwards, above your head if you can, keeping your elbows straight and hands and fingers in line; slowly lower the arms back to the starting position. 5–10 times. *Variation: if one arm is less mobile than the other, clasp your hands together or hold a stick to help the movement at first.*

5. **Two-handed ball throw**. Using both hands, throw a light ball underarm up in the air or against a wall and catch it. 5–10 times. *Variation: use balls of different sizes and weights.*

6. **Gentle press-ups**. Kneeling on your hands and knees on the floor, bend your elbows slightly, with control, to bring your shoulders and chest towards the floor, keeping your head up; straighten your elbows quickly to raise your upper trunk up. 5–10 times.

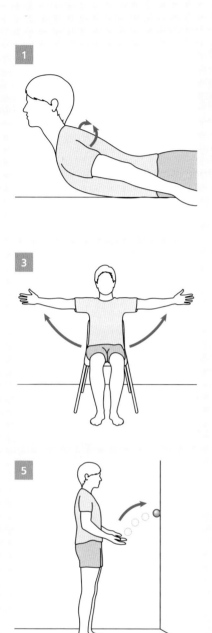

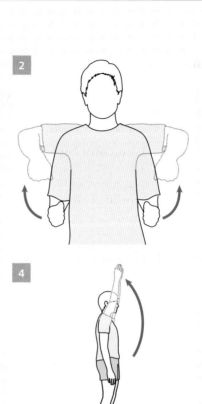

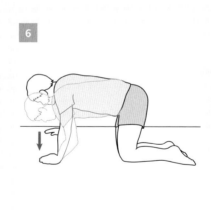

Basic shoulder and upper arm mobilizing and stretching exercises

1. **Gravity-assisted shoulder mobilizer.** Lying on your back, with a soft pillow or small cushion under your head (making sure there is space above and behind your head), clasp your hands together; keeping your elbows straight, lift your arms upwards as far as you can above your head. 10–20 times. *Variation: if it is difficult for you to keep your hands together, hold a bar or stick (e.g. a walking stick) in your hands so that they are shoulder-width apart.*

2. **Gentle flexion-extension shoulder mobilizer.** Standing, bend forwards at the hips so that your trunk is horizontal, and rest one hand on a support; swing your other arm gently backwards and forwards, keeping your elbow straight. 10–20 times.

3. **Gentle rotation shoulder mobilizer.** Standing, bend forwards from the hips, with your trunk horizontal and one hand on a support; keeping your elbow straight, swing the free arm gently round in circles, making the circles as wide as you can. 10–20 times.

4. **Gentle shoulder girdle mobilizer.** Standing, bend forwards from your hips, with your trunk horizontal and one hand on a support; keeping your trunk still, swing your free arm out sideways straightening the elbow, then inwards across your chest letting your elbow bend. 10–20 times.

5. **Shoulder elevation with a pulley.** Rig up a pulley system from a strong fixed point, putting a rope over a bar, branch or strong hook; lift one arm up, extend the other arm downwards and grip the rope; pull down with each hand alternately to lift the other arm to a comfortable limit upwards. 20 times.

6. **Finger wall-climb.** Standing facing a wall, about 15 centimetres (6 inches) away, place one hand on the wall; work your hand upwards using your fingers, to reach as high as you can; when you reach your limit, hold the arm with your other hand, if necessary, to help it reverse the movement. 10–20 times.

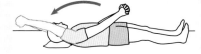

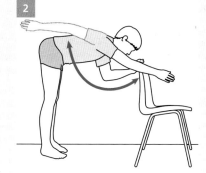

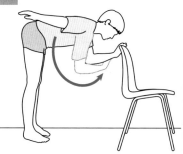

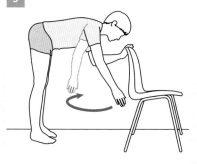

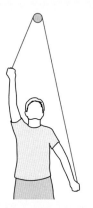

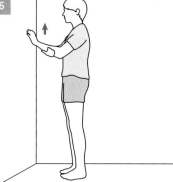

Advanced shoulder and upper arm isometric strengthening exercises

1. Sitting or standing with your arm straight down beside you, sideways on to a wall or a suitable fixed object about 15 centimetres (6 inches) away, press the back of your hand against the wall, keeping your elbow straight; hold for a count of 5, then relax. 3–6 times *Variations: raise your arm forwards and up at varying angles and repeat the isometric pressure against the wall with the back of your hand.*

2. Sitting or standing, lift your arm up forwards and bend your elbow, so that your shoulder and elbow are at right angles; holding the position, press your other hand against the raised hand for a count of 5, then relax. 3–6 times. *Variation: turn the palm of the raised arm forwards, then backwards.*

3. Sitting or standing sideways on to a wall or suitable fixed object, about 8 centimetres (3 inches) away, bend your elbow to a right angle; press the back of your hand against the wall, keeping your elbow by your side; hold for a count of 5, then relax. 3–6 times. *Variation: place your arm forwards and up at varying angles, keeping your elbow bent, and repeat the isometric press with the back of the hand.*

4. Sitting or standing, raise your arm up above your head and bend your elbow to a right angle over the top of your head, palm forwards; press your other palm against the palm of the raised hand and block any movement for a count of 5, then relax. 3–6 times.

5. Sitting or standing, raise your arm up above your head and bend your elbow to a right angle over the top of your head, palm forwards; press your other palm against the back of the raised hand and block any movement for a count of 5, then relax. 3–6 times.

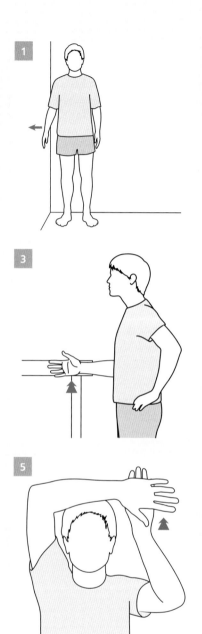

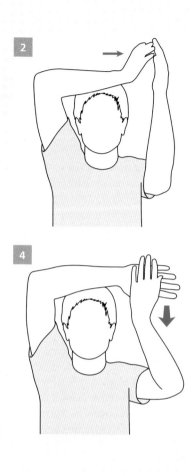

Advanced shoulder and upper arm dynamic strengthening exercises

1. **Arm flexion and medial rotation strengthener**. Lying on your back on the edge of a bed, take your arm over the side of the bed, keeping your elbow straight and your palm up; lift your arm up and across your body diagonally to take your arm across your face, turning your hand inwards and bending your elbow slightly as you raise the arm; reverse the movement with control. 5–10 times.

2. **Arm flexion and lateral rotation strengthener**. Lying on your back, place your arm across your body to the opposite hip, with your elbow straight and palm down; lift your arm upwards and outwards, turning your hand outwards as you lift so that your thumb leads the movement, keeping your elbow straight; reverse the movement with control. 5–10 times.

3. **Shoulder rotation-in-elevation strengthener**. Lying on your back, lift your arm up close to your head, and bend your elbow so that your forearm is above your head, palm facing forwards; keeping your arm in place, move your hand forwards and backwards above your head, twisting the shoulder. 5–10 times, then relax.

4. **One-handed ball throw**. Throw a ball against a wall and catch it with your injured hand. 10–20 times. *Variations: a) throw underarm then overarm; b) increase your distance from the wall; c) vary the size and weight of the ball.*

5. **Quick-fire punches**. Standing with your elbows bent to an acute angle, fists lightly clenched and palms facing upwards, punch the air in front of you rapidly with each arm alternately, turning the fist downwards as your arm goes forwards, and upwards as it returns to the starting position. 20–50 punches with each hand.

1

2

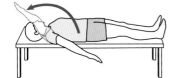

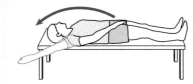

3

4

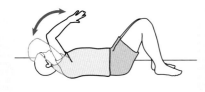

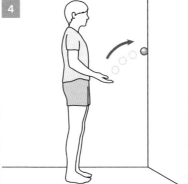

5

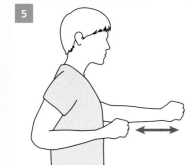

The Shoulder Region and Upper Arm

Advanced shoulder and upper arm mobilizing and stretching exercises

1. **Arm circling**. Standing or sitting, swing your arms round in circles or spirals above your head in an easy continuous rhythm. 10–20 times.

2. **Advanced rotation mobilizer**. Standing, lift one arm, holding the end of a towel or belt, and bend the elbow so that your hand is behind your head; keeping it by your side, bend the other arm behind your back to grasp the other end of the towel or belt; straighten each arm alternately as far as you comfortably can 20 times, then reverse your hand positions and repeat.

3. **Biceps stretch**. Standing up or sitting on a stool, with your back straight, head up, clasp your hands behind your back, palms together; gently lift your arms backwards, keeping your elbows straight, until you feel a gentle stretch over the front of your shoulders and upper arms. Hold for a count of 6, then relax. 5–10 times.

4. **Triceps stretch**. Sitting on a stool or standing up, with your back straight and head up, raise one arm straight up above your head, and bend the elbow so that your hand drops behind your neck; with your other hand, gently pull the raised elbow inwards, towards and slightly behind your head, keeping the elbow well bent. Hold for a count of 6, then relax. 5–10 times.

5. **Shoulder rotation stretch**. Sitting on a stool or standing up, with your back straight and head up, raise one arm up vertically above your head and bend your elbow to drop your hand behind your neck and upper back, palm facing inwards towards your back; keeping the other arm close to your side, bend the elbow so that your hand reaches upwards behind your back, palm facing away from your body; gently press your hands towards each other so that they touch, if possible. Hold for a count of 6, then relax. 5–10 times on each side.

6. **Advanced circumduction mobilizer**. Standing, hold a stick, cord or belt in your hands in front of you; swing the stick in a complete arc over your head to behind your back, keeping your elbows straight, then reverse the movement. 5–10 times. Start with your hands wide apart and gradually bring them closer together.

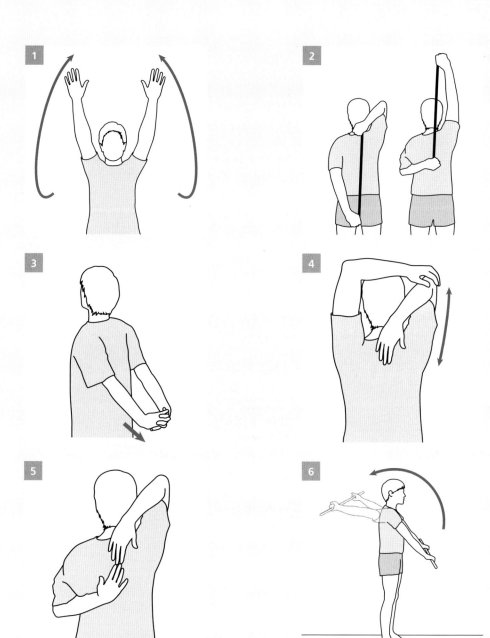

18

The Elbow and Forearm

RIGHT ELBOW, SEEN FROM THE FRONT.

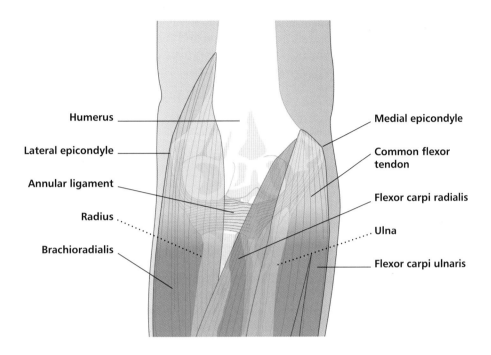

Humerus

Lateral epicondyle

Annular ligament

Radius

Brachioradialis

Medial epicondyle

Common flexor tendon

Flexor carpi radialis

Ulna

Flexor carpi ulnaris

The elbow lies between the humerus (upper arm) and forearm. The forearm, which consists of the radius and ulna bones, connects the elbow to the wrist.

Structure

Bones

The lower end of the humerus spreads out sideways each way, but more on the inner side than the outer. This is why the forearm does not hang vertically when the elbow is straight and your palms facing forwards, but is set at an angle away from the upper arm and the body. This is called the 'carrying angle', and is greater in females than males.

The epicondyles are protrusions on either side of the lower end of the humerus. The medial epicondyle is on the inner (little finger) side of the bone, while the lateral epicondyle is on the outer side (leading down to the thumb). You can feel both epicondyles with your fingers, just above and behind the elbow. The medial epicondyle is also known as the 'funny bone', because the nerve which lies directly behind it causes odd sensations if the bone gets knocked.

The radius is on the outer (thumb) side of the forearm and the ulna on the inner (little finger) side. The head of the radius, just below the elbow, is difficult to feel from the surface, because it is covered with layers of muscles, but at the wrist you can feel the bone's pointed tip or styloid process. The top of the ulna is called the olecranon, which is the prominent bone on the back of the elbow. It forms a spanner shape, with a pointed tip on its top front edge called the olecranon process, and another lower down called the coronoid process. The head of the ulna is at its lower end, with a jutting styloid process on its edge. The ulnar head is visible and palpable when you turn your hand palm down.

Joints

Three bones make up the elbow joint, the humerus, radius and ulna. The elbow joint consists of two parts, one between the end of the humerus and the ulna, the *humeroulnar* part, and the other between the humerus and radius, the *humeroradial* part. Technically it is termed a compound synovial joint. The joint structure creates a triangular hollow called the cubital fossa on the front of the elbow.

At the lower end of the humerus there is a knuckle called the trochlea, which forms the upper part of the humeroulnar joint. To the outer side of the trochlea is a rounded surface called the capitulum, which is the surface for the flattened circular top of the radius in the humeroradial component. Just above the back of the trochlea is a hollow called the olecranon fossa, shaped to receive the olecranon process on the ulna when the elbow is fully straight. On the front of the humerus, just above the trochlea, there is a similar but smaller depression called the coronoid fossa, which receives the coronoid process on the front edge of the ulna when the elbow is fully bent.

The two forearm bones link to each other in the superior (proximal or upper) and inferior (distal or lower) radio-ulnar joints, which are technically uniaxial pivot joints. In the upper joint, the head of the radius abuts on a small recess on the ulna called the radial notch. In the lower joint the radius has an ulnar notch, shaped to receive the edge of the ulnar head.

Capsules, ligaments and bursae

The elbow joint is protected by a capsule which surrounds it completely, and which is lined with a fluid-producing synovial membrane. At either side of the joint are ligaments which prevent sideways movement. The ulnar collateral ligament on the inner side is attached to the medial epicondyle on the humerus and the edge of the top of the ulna. The radial collateral ligament on the outer side is attached not only to the elbow bones, but also to the annular ligament, a strong band which encircles the head of the radius and binds it to the top of the ulna to form the superior radioulnar joint. The radius and ulna are connected down most of their length by an interosseous membrane, which, apart from binding the two bones together, provides a surface for the attachment of the deep forearm muscles. The inferior radioulnar joint is enclosed in a capsule with a synovial membrane lining. There is a fibrocartilaginous disc between the lower ends of the radius and ulna.

Where soft tissues pass close to bones or other soft tissues, they are usually separated by bursae, the most prominent of which lies over the olecranon, separating the bone from the triceps tendon.

Muscles and tendons

Brachialis and the biceps brachii tendon (p. 243) lie over the front of the elbow. The biceps tendon is attached to the radius, with a further attachment to the back of the ulna. Brachialis lies under biceps along the front of the humerus, and forms a tendon at its lower end which fixes to the upper part of the ulnar shaft. Triceps (p. 244) and anconeus are at the back of the elbow. The triceps tendon attaches to the top of the olecranon at the back of the elbow. Anconeus is a triangular muscle which is attached to the back of the lateral epicondyle of the humerus and to triceps at its upper part, and to the side of the olecranon and the back of the top of the ulna lower down.

The common extensor tendon joins the wrist and hand extensor muscles (p. 293) to the lateral epicondyle of the humerus, while the common flexor tendon (p. 292) is attached to the medial epicondyle. Pronator teres has one attachment just above the medial epicondyle and another on the side of the coronoid process, and passes down and across the forearm to attach to the outer side of the radius.

There are several deep-lying muscles attached to the forearm. Supinator arises from the lateral epicondyle, the radial collateral ligament in the elbow and the annular ligament in the superior radioulnar joint, and is attached to the outer side of the upper end of the radius. Abductor pollicis longus extends from the back of the ulnar shaft, radius and interosseous membrane to the base of the thumb. Extensor pollicis brevis, which is closely connected to the thumb abductor, spreads from the back of the radius and interosseous membrane to the base of the thumb. Extensor pollicis longus is attached to the upper part of the ulnar shaft and the interosseous membrane and fixes on to the base of the thumb tip (distal phalanx) at its lower end. Extensor indicis follows a parallel path to attach to the back of the index finger. On the front of the forearm is the deep-lying pronator quadratus muscle, which spreads across the lower parts of the ulna and radius.

MUSCLES AND TENDONS ON THE BACK OF THE RIGHT FOREARM AND HAND.

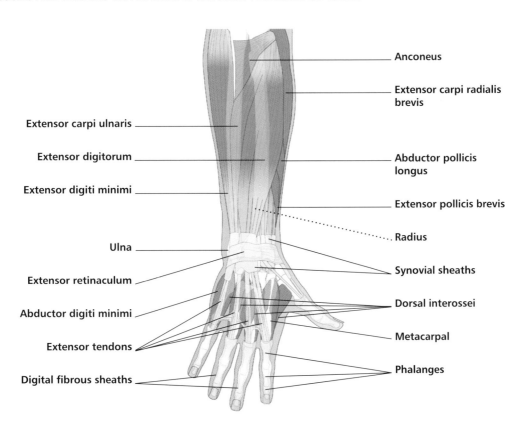

Anconeus

Extensor carpi radialis brevis

Extensor carpi ulnaris

Extensor digitorum

Extensor digiti minimi

Abductor pollicis longus

Extensor pollicis brevis

Radius

Ulna

Synovial sheaths

Extensor retinaculum

Dorsal interossei

Abductor digiti minimi

Metacarpal

Extensor tendons

Phalanges

Digital fibrous sheaths

Functions

The elbow and forearm are crucial to all sports involving the arms, such as racket games, throwing events, archery, fencing, canoeing, rowing, sailing, baseball, cricket, American football, rugby, water polo, volleyball, handball, boxing, the martial arts, wrestling, judo, rock climbing, skiing and weightlifting.

The two parts of the elbow joint work together and are closely linked in structure and function to the superior radioulnar joint. The combined movements allow you to bring your hand to your face or head, and to turn your palm upwards, inwards or downwards when your elbow is bent. When the elbow is straight the mobility of the shoulder allows the hand to be turned at different angles. In people with extremely flexible, hypermobile joints the elbows hyperextend or 'bend backwards' when straightened fully.

The elbow is considered to be a hinge joint. The elbow can bend (flex) and straighten (extend), but there is a slight, imperceptible twisting movement in the ulna during these movements, outwards from the body into supination on bending, and inwards into pronation on straightening. As the radius is not held tightly against its adjacent bones, its head can be moved passively forwards, backwards and sideways. These are accessory movements which you cannot activate consciously.

Working concentrically against gravity or a resistance, brachialis flexes the elbow. It works eccentrically to control the reverse movement under the influence of gravity. Biceps acts with brachialis to bend the elbow, and helps supinator to turn the forearm outwards, if needed. Brachioradialis helps to bend the elbow when extra effort is required, and is at its strongest when the forearm is in mid-position, with the thumb upwards.

Triceps extends the elbow, acting concentrically against gravity or a resistance, helped by anconeus if necessary. They pay out eccentrically to control the opposite movements. Press-ups and dips are exercises which depend on triceps and anconeus strength.

Anconeus may also hold the ulna in place during pronation of the forearm, in which the radius pivots to cross over the ulna, turning the hand palm downwards. The movement of pronation is effected by pronator quadratus, helped by pronator teres when necessary.

Pain and complications

Gradual or unexplained pain and swelling in the elbow can be caused by an inflammatory arthritic condition (p. 12) or an infection (p. 13). Pain can also be referred into the elbow and forearm from the neck (p. 219).

Elbow and forearm injuries

Any of the bones and soft tissues forming the elbow and forearm can be damaged through trauma or overuse at any age. Injury has a direct effect on the upper arm, wrist and hand, and can impair function in the shoulder and upper back on both sides.

Traumatic fracture

The bones of the elbow and forearm can be broken, distorted or cracked through trauma. Fracture can happen together with dislocation, and there may also be nerve or circulatory damage. If a distraction force pulls a tendon away from the bone, the tendon's bony attachment point can be broken off in an avulsion fracture. Loose bodies can form in the elbow following trauma. Fractures can happen at any age. In children fractures are often greenstick, in which one side of the damaged bone breaks, but the other side remains whole and bends. The growth areas can be damaged: the articular epiphyses within the joint area are more likely to be damaged if there is a compressive force on them, while traction forces tend to damage the non-articular epiphyses.

What you feel
There is usually instant pain. The elbow may be distorted, and there may be bleeding. Swelling of the forearm and hand usually follows. Movements are severely limited or impossible because of pain and muscle inhibition. You may notice numbness, tingling or a sensation of cold in your forearm. Shock can set in after the accident. In a minor accident, pain, swelling and stiffness may only become noticeable some time later.

Causes
Fractures can be caused by a fall on to the elbow, forearm or hand, violent wrenching or twisting, or a direct blow to the bones. Your bones are more vulnerable if you suffer from mineral deficiency or a bone condition such as osteoporosis.

Directions
Any fracture must be treated as an emergency, so you should go to hospital as quickly as possible. You may be kept under observation for about three days in case potentially serious problems with your circulation arise. You may need an operation to realign the broken parts of the bone(s) or to remove any loose bone fragments from the elbow. Later, your elbow or forearm may be immobilized in a plaster cast or splint. If the elbow is fixed in the bent position, it is usually supported in a sling. Your wrist may also be immobilized, at least for the first phase of healing, but your fingers will be left free if possible. Rehabilitation to restore function in the elbow is a very gradual, gentle process, to avoid the risk of myositis ossificans (p. 8).

How long?
6–24 months.

Dislocation

The bones of the elbow and forearm can be dislodged from their normal positions by a sudden traumatic force. The ulna can come away from the end of the humerus, while the radial head can be torn out of the annular ligament. A dislocation can happen together with a fracture, and can cause disruption to the circulatory and nerve systems in the injured area. Injury can happen at any age. In children and infants dislocation of the superior radioulnar joint is often referred to as 'pulled elbow'.

What you feel
There is immediate pain, and you cannot move the elbow and forearm normally. There is usually swelling and bruising, and there may be bleeding. The normal contours of the elbow or forearm are distorted. If the radial head has dislocated, the forearm is held blocked in pronation, with the palm facing downwards. If there is nerve involvement, you may feel tingling or numbness down the forearm into your hand. If the circulation is impaired in ischaemia (p. 9), your skin may look an abnormal colour.

Causes
Violent pressure pulls the bones apart or pushes them in abnormal directions. You may have fallen on to your elbow or hand, or your arm may have got trapped while you were moving at speed.

Directions
A dislocation must be treated as an emergency. The bones are usually manipulated back into place, and you may need an operation to mend the soft tissues if they are badly damaged. The elbow and forearm are usually immobilized in a splint or plaster cast which extends to include the hand, although your fingers may be free. Like the treatment for a fracture, rehabilitation is a very gradual process.

How long?
6–24 months.

Bone stress injury

Overuse can cause a stress fracture in any of the bones of the elbow and forearm at any age. In children and teenagers the growth points (apophyses) where tendons are attached can be affected.

What you feel
There is pain associated with a particular activity involving your arm. The pain is usually felt after exercising at first, often at night. If you continue your sport, the pain gradually gets worse. Rest eases it, but it recurs if you resume your sport too soon. There is usually localized tenderness if you press on the affected bone, and you may notice slight swelling, warmth or redness over the painful area.

Causes
Excessive pressure on a bone by repetitive muscle or tendon activity creates micro-damage in the hard substance of the affected bone. You may have started a new sport overenthusiastically, resumed training after a lay-off, or increased your schedule suddenly in preparation for a competition. You may have been training intensively without sufficient recovery time. You are more likely to get a stress fracture if you suffer from mineral deficiency or a bone condition such as osteoporosis.

Directions
As a stress fracture may not show up on an X-ray in the early stages, the diagnosis is usually made on the basis of your description of the pain in relation to your activities. If there is doubt, your doctor may send you for further investigations such as a bone scan or blood tests. Once the stress fracture has been diagnosed, you have to rest from painful activities long enough to allow the crack to heal. To promote healing, you should do alternative training and exercises which do not cause pain. Once the bone has healed, you should allow two more weeks before resuming your normal sport in gradual stages.

How long?
6–16 weeks.

Elbow synovitis

The fluid-filled lining inside the elbow joint can be damaged or irritated, so it produces extra fluid. Sometimes the lining becomes thickened. This is usually because of a traumatic injury, although it can result from cumulative stress. It can happen at any age.

What you feel
The elbow is painful and stiff, and you can see and feel localized swelling. The elbow may feel warm.

Causes
Synovitis can appear as a late reaction to an injury. The elbow may have been bruised by a knock or in a fall. In some cases there is nipping of the synovium through repetitive forceful joint movements. You are more vulnerable to synovitis if you have a family tendency to inflammatory arthritis, or if you have hyperextending elbows.

Directions
You may be given a special splint to prevent further irritation. If the problem is complicated and becomes long-standing, you may be offered an operation.

How long?
3–9 months.

Posterior elbow impingement

Impact between the olecranon and its fossa causes irritation in the joint lining which results in damage to the joint cartilage and underlying bone. Bony spurs can form, especially on the tip of the olecranon, and bone fragments can break off into the joint. This may be a sudden injury, but more often it is an overuse syndrome. It can happen at any age.

What you feel
There is pain at the back of the elbow when you extend the elbow fully, and sometimes on other movements too. There may be local tenderness and swelling. The elbow can become stiff.

Causes
Posterior impingement is a risk in sports involving forceful extension movements, especially tennis, badminton, javelin throwing, baseball pitching, water polo and powerlifting. It is more likely to happen if you have hyperextending elbows.

Directions
To avoid further irritation, the elbow may be splinted in a support which allows normal bending movements but blocks full extension. Exercises will be recommended to correct your elbow biomechanics, focussing especially on isometric strengthening with the elbow bent. If there are bony spurs or loose bodies in the joint, you may be offered an operation.

How long?
3–12 months.

Olecranon bursitis

Any of the bursae around the elbow can be damaged through trauma or overuse. Most commonly affected is the olecranon bursa, and the problem can happen at any age.

What you feel
The bursa becomes enlarged and may feel tender if you press it. Movements which put pressure on the affected bursa cause pain. In olecranon bursitis there is pain when you bend and straighten the elbow, and the movements may become slightly limited.

Causes
Traumatic injury usually results from a hard knock on the back of the elbow. An overuse injury can be caused by friction, perhaps from a tight, hard or badly fitting elbow protector, or through leaning on the elbow for long periods. Infection or food intolerance (p. 11) can be contributory factors. You are more likely to suffer from bursitis if you have a family tendency to gout or inflammatory joint disease (p. 12), or if you have hyperextending elbows.

Directions
You should protect the elbow from friction, and avoid painful activities. A soft elbow support or doughnut-shaped padding can be helpful. You can rub ice, heparinoid cream or arnica round the edges of the bursa. If there is any doubt about what has caused the problem, your doctor will refer you for tests. Fluid may be aspirated (drawn out) from the bursa. If the problem becomes long-standing, you may be offered an injection, or, as a last resort, an operation. If the bursa is removed surgically, a new one normally grows in its place.

How long?
3 weeks to several months.

Soft tissue injuries

The ligaments, tendons and muscles which act on the elbow and forearm can be torn, partly torn or strained through trauma or overuse, at any age. In young children and teenagers, soft tissue injury often happens together with bone damage. In adults traction spurs can form when there is repeated excessive stress from a tendon pulling against a bone.

What you feel
In a traumatic injury there is immediate sudden pain over the damaged area, often with bruising and swelling, whereas pain builds up gradually in an overuse injury. The damaged tissue hurts on movement and direct pressure. Ligament damage may make the elbow feel loose or unstable. An injured muscle or tendon hurts when you contract or stretch it; so, for instance, if the extensor muscles on the back of the forearm are hurt, you have pain if you clench your fist or bend your wrist backwards forcefully, and when you stretch the muscles by bending (flexing) the wrist forwards. You may be aware of localized tightness, and there may be visible muscle wasting in the injured area.

Causes

Damage happens through shearing, traction or compression forces. The ulnar collateral ligament on the inner side of the elbow is particularly vulnerable to sudden abnormal movements which open up the joint and twist it. The tendons and muscles can be damaged through a sudden forceful contraction or stretch, a blocked movement, or cumulatively through excessive repetitive actions.

Directions

When a soft tissue injury has been diagnosed, self-help and treatments are aimed at reducing pain and swelling, and your practitioner will set you exercises to restore flexibility and strength.

How long?

3–12 weeks.

Compartment syndrome

Fluid can build up within a muscle sheath as a result of overuse or trauma in the elbow or forearm, at any age. The pressure of the fluid can cause ischaemia (p. 9) and nerve disruption.

What you feel

Any muscle compartment can be affected, although it is most often the front (palm side) of the forearm. Compartment syndrome of the anconeus causes pain on the outer side of the elbow which mimics 'tennis elbow'. There is continuous pain in the affected area, and you cannot activate the muscles normally. You may also have a feeling of numbness or tingling. Trying to move your elbow, wrist or fingers hurts. There is a tense swelling and your skin may look pale. In a severe case the pulse in your wrist may stop beating and your joint movements can be blocked.

Causes

Acute compartment syndrome can occur apparently spontaneously, but usually follows trauma to the elbow or forearm bones or muscles. Overuse compartment syndrome can result from overtraining in any sport which stresses the elbow and forearm.

Directions

In an acute case you should refer to your doctor or specialist urgently. If decompression surgery (fasciotomy) is needed, it should be done as quickly as possible. If the injury is more minor, you may be given treatment to reduce the swelling and restore strength and mobility to the area. A soft protective support might help.

How long?

6 weeks to 9 months. In rare cases the effects are long-term.

'Tennis elbow'

The common extensor tendon on the outer side of the elbow can be damaged, partly torn or strained through trauma, but more often through overuse. The injury is known technically as lateral epicondylitis. It can happen at any age, but is rare in children. It often happens together with neck problems, and referred symptoms from the neck can seem exactly the same as those of 'tennis elbow'.

What you feel
If the damage is traumatic, you may feel sudden pain over the outer side of your elbow when you activate the extensor tendons by gripping an object or moving your wrist. There is a tender point if you press on it. In an overuse injury there is gradually increasing pain over the lateral epicondyle when the extensor tendons contract or are stretched. The pain can wear off when the arm is warmed up, but it gradually gets worse if you continue the activity which caused it. The bone can become extremely sensitive, your wrist extensor muscles may waste, and your grip may be weakened. Pain on gripping can depend on whether the object is thick or thin, and may vary according to the position of your arm, whether it is straight or bent, raised or down by your side, or stretched forwards or behind you. You may also notice pain or stiffness in your neck or shoulder.

Causes
'Tennis elbow' is not confined to tennis players. Sudden trauma usually involves a blow to the side of the elbow, which can happen in sports like lacrosse, or if you fall and hit your elbow against a hard object. Overuse damage can happen through any sport which involves gripping, including skiing, canoeing, rowing, powerlifting and javelin throwing as well as racket sports. You may have started training or competing more intensively, or changed your technique or your equipment. The injury can be secondary to a previous injury in the elbow, wrist, hand or shoulder.

Directions
A simple strap round the forearm just below the elbow or a more elaborate forearm splint can help relieve pressure on the tendon. Try to identify the cause of the problem. Modify your sports equipment or your technique if you have recently made changes. For racket sports, check whether your racket grip is too thick or narrow, or whether your racket is too light or too heavy in the head.

Your practitioner will identify whether your problem is purely in the elbow, or if your shoulder or neck might be involved, and will set out your treatment and exercise programme accordingly, with special focus on the posterior forearm stretch (p. 288), and often the medial hand strengthener (p. 303). You may be offered an injection, or, as a last resort, an operation.

How long?
10 days to several months.

Radial tunnel syndrome

The posterior interosseous branch of the radial nerve becomes trapped where it passes through a tunnel of soft tissues and lies close to the supinator muscle just below the outer side of the elbow. The injury is also known as resistant tennis elbow. It can happen at any age.

What you feel
Because the posterior interosseous nerve supplies the wrist extensor muscles, the symptoms can seem similar to those of 'tennis elbow', except that the localized pain is felt not on the lateral epicondyle, but slightly lower down. The wrist extensor muscles and supinator may tire easily when they are activated. In a bad case they become noticeably weak, even resulting in a 'dropped wrist', because the extensors cannot apply enough force to cock the wrist.

Causes
The nerve can be injured traumatically by a direct blow, or irritated through excessive repetitive forceful movements involving the wrist. The radial tunnel can become narrow because fibrous tissue has formed following other injuries.

Directions
Try to identify the cause of the problem. A soft support for the elbow may help. If the problem is severe and long-standing, you may be offered an operation.

How long?
Usually several weeks.

'Golfer's elbow'

In 'golfer's elbow', technically medial epicondylitis, the common flexor tendon on the inner side of the elbow becomes partly torn, strained or inflamed. This is usually an overuse injury, although it can happen through sudden trauma. It is often associated with neck or shoulder problems. Nerve pain radiating from the neck can cause symptoms that mimic those of 'golfer's elbow'. It can happen at any age, but is rare in children.

What you feel
There is pain over the inner side of the elbow when the common flexor tendon is activated or stretched. Flexing the wrist, gripping and turning the hand inwards towards the little finger side all cause pain. The pain may radiate down the forearm towards the wrist. The inflamed area feels tender to touch. The muscles on the inner (little finger) side of the front of your forearm might waste, and your grip becomes weak.

Causes
In a traumatic injury there may be a direct blow over the common flexor tendon, or a sudden wrench causing stress at its attachment point. Most often 'golfer's elbow' arises through repetitive activities. You may be new to your sport, or have restarted after a lay-off. You may have been training more intensively than normal, or changed your technique or equipment. The injury can follow a problem in your hand, shoulder or neck.

Directions
Correct or discard any equipment which has contributed to the problem. You may need to rethink your technique. Your practitioner will recommend remedial exercises, especially the anterior forearm stretch (p. 288) and the medial hand strengthener (p. 303).

How long?
1 week to 4 months.

Ulnar nerve entrapment

The ulnar nerve can be trapped or compressed in the cubital tunnel at the back of the inner side of the elbow, where the 'funny bone' is. It can also be compressed in the hand (p. 299). Sometimes the compression affects both areas, but more often only one. The nerve becomes damaged and irritated, and the injury is termed a neuropathy. It is usually an overuse syndrome, but can happen through trauma. It can happen at any age.

What you feel
There may be numbness or tingling down the inner side of the forearm, and especially in the ring and little fingers. Your grip may weaken, and you may find it difficult to use the fourth and fifth fingers normally. The symptoms are usually worse when the elbow is bent, especially if you hold it still for a while. At night the fingers may 'go dead' if you sleep on your bent arm. If the problem develops to a severe stage, the muscles of the inner side of the forearm and hand waste, losing their fleshy contour.

Causes
A traumatic injury can result from a direct blow to the nerve at the back of the elbow. Sometimes the nerve is compressed as the result of a fracture. As an overuse syndrome, compression can arise if you tend to lean on your bent elbow for long periods. Faulty technique in sports which involve complex elbow movements, such as javelin throwing, can be a cause. Ulnar nerve compression can be a late effect following some other injury of the elbow which has caused joint swelling or the formation of a bony spur on the edge of one of the bones.

Directions
Correct your posture or sports technique, as appropriate. It may help to use a soft splint to keep your elbow straight, especially at night. Treatment is aimed at controlling the symptoms, improving the circulation through the whole arm and restoring function in the hand and elbow. As a last resort you may be offered an operation to decompress the nerve.

How long?
6 weeks to several months.

Pronator syndrome

The median nerve becomes trapped, irritated or damaged where it lies between the two heads of pronator teres. The same nerve can be compressed further down its course towards the hand, most frequently in the carpal tunnel (p. 299). The injury can happen at any age, but is rare in children.

What you feel
There is a deep ache along the front of the forearm when you contract the pronator muscle, and you may notice tingling or numbness affecting the thumb, index and middle fingers and part of the ring finger. If you press hard on to your forearm in the right place, you can reproduce your pain and symptoms. Gripping an object causes pain, especially if you twist your forearm as well. Your grip may get progressively weaker.

Causes
Compression usually follows injury to the forearm muscles caused by forceful or excessive repetitive movements.

Directions
You may be advised to use a soft support. Your practitioner is likely to recommend exercises to stretch the forearm and correct the balance of muscles around the area. If your case is severe, you may be offered an operation to relieve the pressure on the nerve.

How long?
3–12 months.

Myositis ossificans

Calcification or the formation of particles of bone occurs in the muscles around the joint following an injury which has caused internal bleeding (haematoma).

What you feel
There is increasing stiffness in the joint, possibly with a visible hard swelling. There may or may not be pain.

Causes
The exact reason why some people get this problem is not known. It usually follows an injury which has caused deep bruising or internal bleeding around the elbow joint. Aggressive, forceful massage, manipulations or movements can contribute.

Directions
The joint needs to be rested and protected from any painful or forcible movements. Any treatment must be very gentle and non-invasive. You need to maintain good overall body condition, but avoid any exercises which stress the elbow. Surgery is a last resort. The extra bone tends to re-form if it is removed too soon surgically, often causing increasing blockage in the joint, so surgery is usually not considered until at least a year after the problem has started. Even then there is a risk of recurrence.

How long?
This is a long-term problem.

Elbow osteoarthritis (osteoarthrosis)

The cartilage surfaces over the bone ends in the elbow degenerate, causing loss of joint space and sometimes loose bodies which break off into the joint. The normal contour of the elbow can become deformed. There may also be nerve pressure due to joint or tissue swelling. The problem mainly occurs in later middle age, but can happen to younger adults.

What you feel
However bad the degeneration in the joint, it does not necessarily cause pain. If it does, pain usually occurs when you are using the elbow, especially for forceful movements or under heavy load. The elbow may creak or catch when you move it, and there may be visible swelling and abnormal warmth in the joint. There may be pain at night, sometimes with tingling or numbness down to your fingers. There is increasing stiffness in the joint, with weakening of the surrounding muscles. It can become increasingly bent in fixed flexion deformity.

Causes
Osteoarthritis is often the late result of an injury, especially if you failed to regain full strength and mobility in the joint at the time. Sometimes degeneration occurs through long-term overstressing of the joint, for instance if you have played a racket sport for many years. You are more likely to get the condition if you have a family history of osteoarthritis.

Directions
Use a soft support or protective splint for the elbow if necessary. Your practitioner will recommend exercises to improve movement, stability and strength at the elbow. If the pain is disabling, you may be offered surgery: in the earlier stages this might involve simply cleaning debris or loose bodies out the joint through arthroscopy (keyhole surgery), while later on there may be a case for total elbow replacement.

How long?
This is a long-term condition.

Rehabilitation and recovery

Acute phase

Use the circulatory care measures (p. 27). Your practitioner will tell you which movements you can safely do. You should try to keep your shoulder moving, if possible lifting your arm up at frequent intervals, especially if you have to use a sling for support during the day. If your wrist and fingers are free, you should exercise them too. Alternative training for the unaffected parts of your body should start as soon as possible (p. 25).

Early phase

Your practitioner will compose the programme of exercises according to your injury. After a fracture or dislocation, you might start with isometric exercises and gentle mobilizing movements. For a soft tissue injury, stretching and mobilizing are usually combined with isometric and simple dynamic strengthening exercises. If your injury involved the back of the elbow, especially if you have hyperextending elbows, the emphasis may be on the isometric exercises with the elbow bent, to create better biomechanical balance in the joint. In all cases the elbow and forearm exercises may be combined with the basic wrist and hand strengthening (p. 302), stretching and mobilizing (p. 304) exercises.

Recovery phase

For any major elbow injury, progression through the rehabilitation process is cautious, to avoid the risk of myositis ossificans. Once you have recovered localized strength and a good range of movement, you can use light weights for the dynamic strengthening exercises, gradually increasing the load. The exercises can be combined with the advanced strengthening exercises for the wrist and hand (p. 306) and dynamic shoulder exercises (p. 264). You should not progress to the final recovery phase (p. 308) before your elbow and forearm are fully mobile, strong and pain-free on all movements.

Isometric elbow and forearm exercises with elbow flexed

1. **Elbow flexion, forearm supinated**. Sit at a table with your arm by your side, elbow bent to a right angle and your hand palm up against the underside of the table; press your hand upwards against the table; hold the contraction for a count of 5, then relax completely. 3–6 times. *Variation: press with the thumb side of your hand as well, as if trying to turn the hand over, to include isometric pronation activity.*

2. **Elbow flexion, forearm in mid-position**. Sit at a table with your arm by your side, elbow bent to a right angle, hand turned midway so the thumb is uppermost and placed against the underside of the table; press up against the table with the edge of your hand; hold for a count of 5, then relax. 3–6 times.

3. **Elbow flexion, forearm pronated**. Sit at a table with your arm by your side, elbow bent to a right angle, hand palm down, and the back of your hand against the underside of the table; press upwards with the back of your hand against the underside of the table; hold for a count of 5, then relax. 3–6 times. *Variation: press with the thumb side of your hand as well, as if trying to turn the hand over, to include isometric supination activity.*

4. **Triceps action, forearm pronated**. Sit at a table with your arm by your side, elbow bent to a right angle, and hand palm down on the table; press your hand down against the table top; hold for a count of 5, relax. 3–6 times.

5. **Triceps action, forearm supinated**. Sit at a table with your arm by your side, elbow bent to a right angle and hand palm up, resting on the table; press the back of your hand down against the table top; hold for a count of 5, relax. 3–6 times. *Variations for exercises 1–5: sit closer to the table, then further away, to alter the elbow angle. This changes the muscle work from mid-range to inner then outer range.*

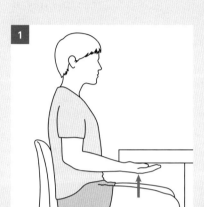

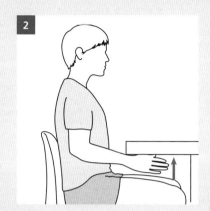

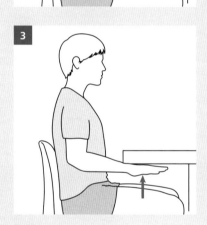

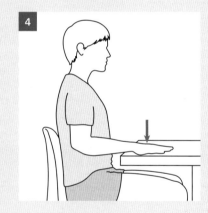

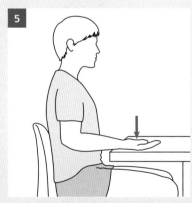

Dynamic elbow and forearm strengthening exercises

1. **Biceps curl**. Sitting with your with your head up, back supported, arm straight down by your side and palm facing forwards, bend your elbow to bring your hand up to the front of your shoulder, keeping your upper arm still; slowly reverse the movement. 5–10 times.

2. **Brachialis strengthener**. Sitting with your with your head up, back supported, arm straight down by your side and palm facing backwards, bend your elbow to bring the back of your hand up to the front of your shoulder, keeping your upper arm still; slowly reverse the movement. 5–10 times.

3. **Triceps strengthener, prone-lying**. Lying on your front at the edge of a bed, with your upper arm supported, bend your elbow to lower your forearm over the side of the bed, palm facing downwards; straighten your elbow fully, keeping your upper arm still; slowly reverse the movement. 5–10 times.

4. **Triceps strengthener, upright**. Sitting or standing, lift your arm up close to your head, and drop your hand behind your neck; keeping the upper arm still, straighten your elbow to lift your hand in the air. Bend and straighten the elbow 5–10 times.

5. **Pronation and supination strengthener**. Sit with your arm by your side, elbow bent to a right angle, forearm unsupported, a light weight in your hand and palm facing down; turn your hand so that your palm faces upwards, keeping your upper arm still, then reverse the movement with control. 5–10 times.

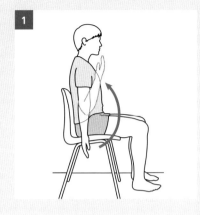

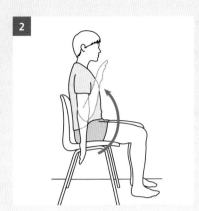

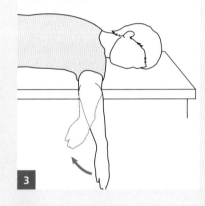

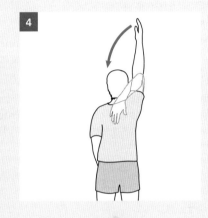

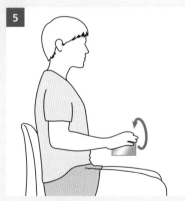

Elbow and forearm stretching and mobilizing exercises

1. **Early elbow flexion and extension mobilizer**. Sitting or lying with a pillow under your arm, use your other hand to bend and straighten the elbow very gently – do not force the movement. 5–20 times.

2. **Elbow flexion and extension mobilizer, lying down**. Lying on your back with your arm by your side, gently bend and straighten your elbow as much as you can. 10–20 times.

3. **Posterior forearm stretch**. Sit or stand with your upper arm by your side and your forearm just in front of you, palm down, fist closed, wrist flexed and elbow bent to about 45 degrees; press the back of your hand gently with your other hand to feel a slight pull on the muscles on the back of the forearm; hold for a count of 6, then relax. 5–10 times. *Variation: hold your wrist and elbow at different angles.*

4. **Anterior forearm stretch**. Sit or stand with your arm held straight out in front of you, fingers extended and palm up; keeping your outstretched arm in place, use the other hand to press your palm backwards, extending the wrist, so that you feel a slight pull on the muscles on the front of the forearm; hold for a count of 6, then relax. 5–10 times.

5. **Pronation and supination mobilizer**. Sit or stand with your arm by your side, elbow bent to a right angle, holding a stick or light racket in your hand; gently turn your hand inwards and outwards, keeping your upper arm still. 10–20 times.

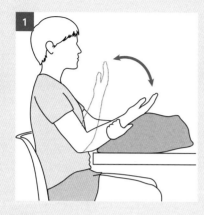

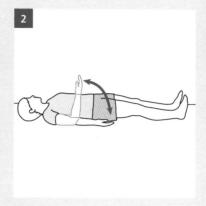

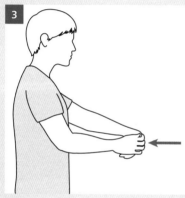

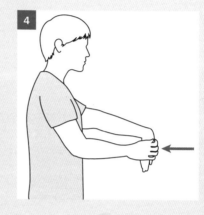

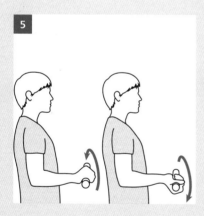

19

The Wrist and Hand

RIGHT WRIST AND HAND, SEEN FROM THE FRONT.

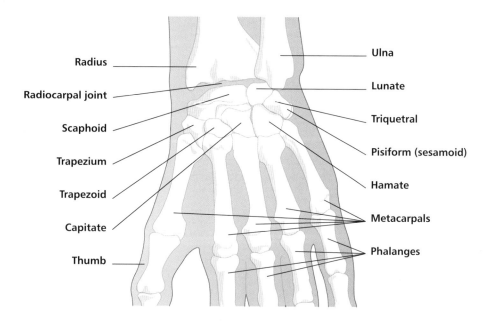

Radius

Radiocarpal joint

Scaphoid

Trapezium

Trapezoid

Capitate

Thumb

Ulna

Lunate

Triquetral

Pisiform (sesamoid)

Hamate

Metacarpals

Phalanges

The wrist or carpus links the hand to the forearm. The hand is the end point of the arm or upper limb.

Structure

Bones

The wrist consists of eight small bones arranged in two rows: the scaphoid, lunate, triquetral and pisiform form the upper (proximal) row, abutting on the forearm bones, while the lower (distal) row consists of the trapezium, trapezoid, capitate and hamate, which link to the hand's metacarpal bones.

The hand consists of five metacarpal bones, and fourteen finger bones, or phalanges. The thumb, or pollex, consists of two finger bones, while the four fingers have three each. The bones are numbered from the thumb side. The knuckles on the back of your hand are the expanded ends of the metacarpal bones.

Joints

The bones of the wrist and hand form a series of joints bound by ligaments, muscles and tendons, encased in capsules lined with synovial membranes.

The main wrist joint, or radiocarpal joint, is formed between the end of the radius and the scaphoid, lunate and triquetral. The lower ends of the radius and ulna are bound by a fibrocartilaginous articular disc, which forms an integral part of the wrist joint.

Intercarpal joints link the carpals, and carpometacarpal (CMC) joints lie between the distal row of carpals and the metacarpals. The first carpometacarpal joint, on the thumb side of the wrist, is a sellar (saddle) joint, and is more complicated than the others. The hand joins the fingers at the metacarpophalangeal (MCP) joints. The fingers form proximal interphalangeal (PIP) joints nearest the hand, with the distal interphalangeal (DIP) joints leading to the fingertips.

Muscles and tendons

The main muscles and tendons which control the wrist extend from the elbow into the hand, with some reaching almost to the ends of the fingers. The hand is controlled by long muscles from the forearm which are attached to the various hand bones, and by small muscles called the intrinsics which lie in between the hand bones. Where tendons cross over each other or other tissues, they are enclosed in synovial sheaths which provide protection and lubrication for frictionless movement.

FLEXOR MUSCLES OF THE RIGHT FOREARM AND WRIST, SEEN FROM THE FRONT.

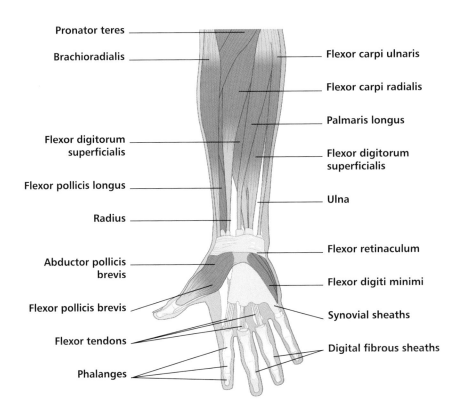

On the front, or palm side, of the wrist and hand are the flexor muscles: flexor carpi radialis, palmaris longus, flexor carpi ulnaris and flexor digitorum superficialis. They are attached at their upper end mainly to the common flexor tendon at the inner side of the elbow (p. 271). The finger tendons are held in place over the front of the wrist bones by a thickened ligament called the flexor retinaculum, which forms the carpal tunnel.

On the back of the wrist and hand are the extensors: extensor carpi radialis longus, extensor carpi radialis brevis, extensor digitorum, extensor digiti minimi and extensor carpi ulnaris. These arise mainly from the common extensor tendon on the outer side of the elbow, and are held down at the wrist by the extensor retinaculum.

Muscles which lie more deeply in the forearm include flexor digitorum profundus and flexor pollicis longus on the front, and abductor pollicis longus, extensor pollicis longus, extensor pollicis brevis and extensor indicis on the back.

The thenar eminence forms the raised pad on the thumb side of the palm, and the hypothenar eminence on the little finger side. The thenar muscles consist of abductor pollicis brevis, opponens pollicis and flexor pollicis, while the hypothenar eminence comprises palmaris brevis, abductor digiti minimi, flexor digiti minimi brevis and opponens digiti minimi. The other intrinsics, which connect the metacarpals to the thumb and fingers, are the adductor pollicis, the palmar and dorsal interossei and the lumbricals.

MUSCLES AND TENDONS ON THE BACK OF THE RIGHT FOREARM AND HAND.

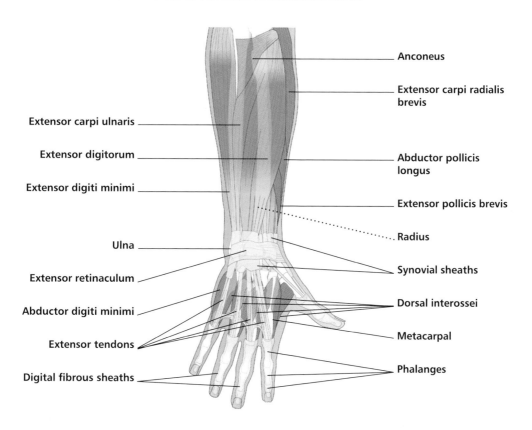

Functions

The wrist and hand coordinate with the forearm, elbow, arm and shoulder. You can perform delicate movements like writing, sewing and playing an instrument or darts, and you can scratch your back or do up zips behind you. The fingers, hands, wrists and arms develop special strength for activities like handstands, rock climbing, archery, volleyball, racket sports, throwing events and martial arts.

Wrist movements

The radiocarpal, intercarpal and carpometacarpal joints all work together. The wrist can bend forwards (flex), bringing the palm of the hand towards the forearm. Against gravity, the superficial flexors of the forearm act concentrically to perform the movement, helped by the deep flexor muscles if necessary, and pay out eccentrically to control the wrist as it straightens out again. The opposite movement of extension is performed by the superficial extensor muscles acting concentrically against gravity, helped by the deep extensors.

The wrist can also bend from side to side: into adduction or ulnar deviation when the movement is towards the little finger side of the hand; and into abduction or radial deviation towards the thumb side. Adduction is performed by flexor and extensor carpi ulnaris. Abduction is more limited, and is performed by flexor carpi radialis and the extensors carpi radialis longus and brevis, helped by abductor pollicis longus and extensor pollicis brevis.

Circling the wrist in either direction is a combination of all the wrist's movements.

Hand and finger movements

The metacarpophalangeal joints allow for flexion, extension, adduction and abduction. Flexion is freest: you can bend the second to fifth metacarpophalangeal joints to about 90°, the first, at the thumb, slightly less. The intrinsic lumbricals and interossei take a lead in flexing the MCP joints: the palmar interossei adduct the fingers, bringing them towards the middle finger when the fingers are held straight; the dorsal interossei abduct the fingers, moving them away from the middle finger.

The PIP and DIP finger joints bend, bringing the fingers towards the palm of the hand, mainly through the action of the long flexor muscles. The lumbricals and interossei, helped by the finger extensors, straighten the fingers.

The thumb moves across the palm mainly through the action of opponens pollicis and flexor pollicis brevis, helped by adductor pollicis and flexor pollicis longus when you need to exert more pressure. Abductores pollicis brevis and longus move the thumb outwards. To bend the thumb, you use flexor pollicis brevis and opponens pollicis, together with flexor pollicis longus if the thumb's MCP and IP joints are also flexed. Extending the thumb involves abductor pollicis longus and extensores pollicis longus and brevis.

The thumb gives you grip, whether with the whole hand or in a pincer between the thumb and a finger. Grip is strongest when the wrist is cocked or extended, and weakened if the wrist is bent.

Pain and complications

Unexplained or unusual pain and swelling in the wrist and hand can be caused by inflammatory joint disease such as rheumatoid arthritis, circulatory problems, infection, food intolerance (p. 11), reflex sympathetic dystrophy (p. 10), or it can be referred from the elbow, shoulder or neck. Very rarely, there might be bone disease, including a tumour.

Wrist and hand injuries

The bones and soft tissues of the wrist and hand can be damaged through trauma or overuse at any age. Injury has a direct effect on the wrist and forearm on the same side, and can impede function in the upper arm, shoulder and upper back.

Traumatic fracture

A traumatic accident can cause a break or crack in any of the wrist or hand bones. There can be joint dislocation as well. Sometimes the bony attachment point of a ligament is broken off in an avulsion fracture. Wrist fractures mostly involve the end of the radius. In a Colles' fracture the end of the radius breaks and the wrist is displaced backwards. Traumatic injury can happen at any age. Radial and ulnar fractures in children often involve the epiphyses or growth plates of the bones at the wrist.

What you feel
There may be immediate pain, or surprisingly little. Pain may come on or increase some time after the accident. If the bones are displaced, there is visible deformity. There may be bleeding, swelling and/or bruising. If there is nerve damage as well, you may feel tingling or numbness in your wrist and hand. As the bone heals, you may feel a deep aching in it, and the bone may feel enlarged.

Causes
There can be direct force, as in a fall on to the hand, or shearing or wrenching if your hand gets caught and pulled. Bones fracture more easily if you have mineral deficiency or bone disease such as osteoporosis.

Directions
Your wrist and hand should be protected with firm but soft bandaging in the first instance, and your arm supported in a sling. You need to be assessed and treated immediately in the casualty department. Your wrist may be immobilized in a splint or plaster cast (see image right). If the bones are displaced, they may be manipulated back in a reduction of the fracture. In some cases surgery may be advised.

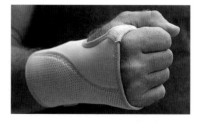

Fractures in the small bones of the wrist, especially the scaphoid, can be difficult to identify on X-ray: if you have continuing pain, you should refer back to your specialist in case the diagnosis was missed.

How long?
6–18 months.

Stress fracture

The bones of the wrist, especially the end of the radius and the scaphoid, can be cracked through overload and overuse. Stress fractures in the hand are rare, but can happen, especially in the metacarpal bones. A stress fracture in the wrist or hand can happen at any age.

What you feel
There is aching or pain after exercising at first, often at night. The pain gradually gets worse if you continue your activities. The affected bone hurts if you press on it. There may be some swelling, and a feeling of warmth over the painful spot. Wrist or hand movements can become stiff and limited.

Causes
Overload is related to doing too much repetitive training, putting excessive strain on the tendons and bones, without allowing enough rest days between sessions. You are more likely to suffer a stress fracture if a previous injury has weakened the wrist muscles or created imbalance, or if you have mineral deficiency or bone disease such as osteoporosis.

Directions
You have to rest from any painful activities for as long as it takes for the bone to mend fully. Meanwhile, you should do alternative exercises to stimulate the circulation and promote healing. The wrist and hand may be protected in a splint in the first instance. In certain circumstances you may be offered an operation. Allow two more weeks after healing before gradually resuming your sport.

How long?
3–12 months.

Kienböck's disease

The lunate bone in the wrist is damaged when its blood supply is impaired. The bone substance gradually deteriorates in a process called avascular necrosis or osteonecrosis (p. 9).

What you feel
The wrist hurts or aches, and usually becomes swollen. The bone is tender if you press on it. Turning the hand palm upwards, supinating the forearm, hurts. The wrist becomes increasingly stiff, with limited flexion and extension. Your grip weakens.

Causes
Kienböck's condition can follow trauma or overuse injury in the wrist, but often the exact cause is not known. It is thought that some people are vulnerable to the problem from birth. In some cases the lunate is served by only one artery instead of the normal two. Some people have a discrepancy in the length of their forearm bones: having a relatively short ulna or long radius is thought to contribute to Kienböck's disease.

Directions
The wrist is usually protected in a splint or cast. Treatment is aimed at improving the blood supply and reducing pain and swelling. If the problem persists, you may be offered an operation.

How long?
8 weeks to several months.

Soft tissue injury

The ligaments, tendons, muscles and other soft tissues in the wrist or hand can be torn, partly torn or strained through trauma or overuse. Injury can happen at any age.

What you feel
In a traumatic accident there may be immediate sharp pain, while overuse injury usually causes slight pain at first, which gradually gets worse. Pain is felt when you move the wrist or use the hand, and the area is tender if you press on it. If there is ligament damage, the wrist or hand may feel unstable. When a tendon or muscle is injured, there is pain when it is contracted or stretched. There may be bleeding, bruising and swelling. If there is nerve involvement, you may experience tingling or numbness in part of the hand. Often the injured area feels warm to the touch.

Causes
Trauma includes a fall on to the hand, or a wrench or shearing strain. Overuse injuries can happen through overtraining or faulty technique in sports which stress the wrists and hands.

Directions
Usually the hand is supported in bandaging or a splint, brace or cast. If there is a major tear, you may be offered an operation. In most cases you will be advised to start moving the wrist and hand gently within pain limits as soon as possible after the injury. If faulty technique or equipment were factors, correct them before resuming your sport fully.

How long?
3–9 months.

Tenosynovitis

The synovial sheaths over the tendons in the wrist and lower end of the forearm can become inflamed through overuse. When this happens at the side of the wrist below the thumb, it is called De Quervain's syndrome. Tenosynovitis can happen at any age, but is more common in adults than in children. Men seem to get tenosynovitis at the back of the wrist more than women, whereas women are more prone to De Quervain's syndrome.

What you feel
A gradual ache develops over the affected tendons, coupled with localized swelling. There is pain on movements which make the tendons contract or stretch, including gripping, but usually none if the wrist and hand are still. The swelling may feel warm to the touch, and can become reddened. There is a characteristic grating feeling and a creaking sound called crepitus when the wrist moves.

Causes
Overdoing repetitive movements is the most common cause, as can happen during rowing training or tennis practice, especially if you have changed your technique or equipment. Sometimes the problem is associated with an infection or an inflammatory arthritic condition.

Directions
Usually the wrist is rested in a removable splint, so that you can use your hand without irritating the tendons. In a chronic case you may be offered medicines, an injection or an operation. Correct your technique or equipment as necessary.

How long?
2 weeks to 3 months.

Ganglion (ganglion cyst)

A localized swelling appears as a soft or hard lump, most often on the back of the wrist, but also elsewhere, including the base of the fingers on the palm side. The lump contains synovial fluid which may have leaked out of one of the wrist joints or from a tendon's synovial sheath. With time the fluid tends to harden. Ganglia can happen at any age, but are more common in adults than children.

What you feel
A ganglion cyst is often painless, even if it is large and unsightly. If painful, it may hurt to stretch the affected area or put direct pressure on it. You may find it increasingly difficult to use your wrist and hand normally.

Causes
The exact cause of ganglia is not known, but they are usually associated with activities which stress the wrist and hand repetitively.

Directions
Often the ganglion subsides if you rest your hand in a splint. Otherwise your doctor might aspirate (drain) it, or it may be excised surgically.

How long?
2 weeks to 6 months.

Nerve damage

Nerves in the wrist and hand can be severed or compressed in traumatic or overuse injuries. Most commonly affected are the median and ulnar nerves. Compression of the median nerve where it passes under the flexor retinaculum on the front of the wrist is an overuse injury known as carpal tunnel syndrome. The ulnar nerve on the inner side of the palm is usually damaged where it passes through a channel called Guyon's canal. Nerve damage can happen at any age, but is least common in young children.

What you feel
When a nerve is severed, you lose both feeling and the ability to control the muscles in the area which it normally supplies. In carpal tunnel syndrome there is pain, sometimes with tingling and numbness, in the palm and fingers on the thumb side of the hand. Pressure on the front of the wrist just below the palm causes pain, for instance when you hold a tennis racket or bicycle handlebars. There may be pain when the hand is clenched, as in writing or throwing darts. You may also have pain at night. The hand muscles can become weak and visibly wasted. In ulnar nerve entrapment the symptoms affect the inner side of the hand and the ring and fifth fingers.

Causes
A nerve can be severed in an accident which results in a deep cut in the wrist or hand. A heavy blow can cause traumatic compression of a nerve, leading to entrapment. Overuse injuries to the median and ulnar nerves are associated with sports or activities which place consistent strain on the wrist and hand. Ulnar nerve entrapment is often caused by gripping tightly for long periods, holding the handlebars of a racing bicycle, for example. Long-term use of crutches can cause pressure on the nerves in the hand. If axillary crutches are used incorrectly (p. 32), pressure on the nerves in the armpit can cause symptoms including numbness and weakness, and even temporary paralysis, in the hands.

Factors which can contribute to or complicate carpal tunnel syndrome include hormonal changes during or after pregnancy, diabetes and hypothyroidism.

Directions
The wrist is usually immobilized in a splint to allow the inflammation to settle. Put padding over any objects which you have to grip. If you have been using crutches, adjust them to reduce pressure on your hands or arms. If your symptoms persist, you may be offered an injection or surgery.

How long?
6 weeks to several months.

Repetitive strain injury (RSI)

Pain develops in the wrist or hand, usually gradually, sometimes on both sides. There may be no specific damage, or tendons or muscles may be strained. There may be nerve involvement. The problem can happen at any age.

What you feel
Repetitive activities involving the wrist and hand are painful. The muscles can become weak and wasted, diminishing your grip strength. You may also have pain around your neck and shoulder, which radiates down your arm.

Causes
RSI is associated with using the hands for repetitive movements while sitting still in poor posture for long periods, especially using a computer.

Directions
Usually the wrist is protected in a brace or splint, and you are prescribed exercises to help your posture and circulation. Physical treatments and exercises usually include the whole arm, shoulder, shoulder girdle and neck. If your problem persists, you may be referred to a specialist for detailed tests. In most cases this is not necessary.

How long?
2 weeks to several months.

Dupuytren's contracture

A knotted tight band of connective tissue forms in your palm, pulling on your fingers, usually the fourth and fifth. The fingers gradually become fixed in flexion. The problem can happen in one or both hands, and affects mainly men in middle or older age. Sometimes a similar syndrome, called Ledderhose disease, affects the feet at the same time.

What you feel
The first sign is usually a painless thickening in the skin of your palm, which gradually gets tighter and forms a knot or lump somewhere in its length. The skin puckers and the affected fingers are pulled downwards into the palm. It becomes increasingly difficult to straighten the fingers or use the hand normally.

Causes
The exact cause is not known. It is not related to physical activities. The condition often runs in families. Diabetes, cigarettes and alcohol make you more vulnerable to it.

Directions

Do not try to straighten out the palm and fingers forcibly as this tends to make the problem worse, but try to maintain strength and mobility through gentle exercises. Avoid tight gripping, and build up the handles on equipment such as tennis rackets and golf clubs. You may be offered needling treatments to cut through the tight cord, or injections to soften it. Otherwise surgery may be an option.

How long?

This is a long-term problem.

Osteoarthritis (osteoarthrosis)

Any of the joints between the bones of the wrist and hand can suffer from progressive wear-and-tear damage to the cartilage covering of the bones. One or both hands can be affected. Osteoarthritis mostly affects people in late middle age or older.

What you feel

The first sign can be night pain or a feeling of increasing stiffness. Pain then develops on using the wrist or hand, which gets worse gradually or sometimes suddenly. Pain can vary with the weather, due to barometric pressure changes. There may also be swelling, a feeling of warmth, and sometimes visible deformity.

Causes

Osteoarthritis is often the result of previous injury, even from many years before. It is more likely to happen if you did not recover full function and balance in the hand at the time. In some cases osteoarthritis develops because of excessive use of your hand(s) and wrist(s) in your job or sport over many years. You may have a family tendency to the condition. Symptoms can be exacerbated by food intolerance reactions (p. 11).

Directions

If the pain is acute, you may need to use a brace or splint for a time, until it settles. If the problem becomes severely disabling, you may be offered an operation.

How long?

This is a long-term condition.

Rehabilitation and recovery

Acute phase

Use the circulatory care measures (p. 27), especially if you have an operation or if your wrist and hand are immobilized in a cast. Your practitioner will tell you which movements you can safely do. In principle, you should keep your shoulder and elbow moving as much as possible. If your fingers are free you should exercise them too. Alternative training for the unaffected parts of your body should start as soon as possible (p. 25).

Early phase

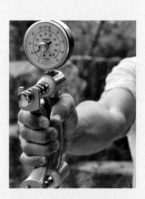

Exercises for the hand's small muscles are usually the first priority, as in the basic strengthening exercises. These are combined, as appropriate, with stretching and mobilizing. Aim to do three to five sessions a day. Your practitioner may measure your grip strength at intervals with a grip dynamometer (see image right) as an objective guide to progress. The exercises should be combined as possible with elbow exercises (p. 286), and basic strengthening and mobility for the shoulder (pp. 258–260), back (pp. 230, 234), abdominals (pp. 190–191) and pelvis (pp. 180–181). You should also work on your legs.

Recovery phase

Once you have recovered fine control and a good of range of movement in the wrist and hand you can progress to the advanced strengthening exercises, using increasing weight resistance where appropriate. You should do the stretching and mobilizing exercises before and after any other types of exercise.

You must recover full strength, mobility and coordination before progressing to the final recovery phase (p. 308) and resuming activities which stress the wrist and hand.

Basic wrist and hand strengthening exercises

1. **Finger extension with adduction and abduction**. Rest your hand palm down on a flat surface, with your fingers slightly spread; lift one finger up, move it from side to side 3 times, then slowly return to the starting position, keeping the palm down throughout; repeat with each finger in turn. 5–10 times.

2. **Pinch grip strengthener**. Press the tips of your thumb and index finger together; hold for a count of 5, then relax. Repeat pressing the thumb against the tip of each finger in turn. 3–6 times.

3. **Hand intrinsic strengthener**. Place your hand flat on a surface, palm down with your fingers slightly spread; keeping your wrist down, fingers and thumb straight and in contact with the surface, draw your fingers and thumb inwards and together so that your knuckles rise and your hand forms an inverted V shape; return to the starting position. 5–10 times.

4. **Fingertip strengthener**. Place your hand on a flat surface, with the palm and fingertips in contact with the surface, finger knuckles bent and lifted up; keeping the palm and fingertips in contact with the surface, bend and straighten the end (DIP) joint of the index finger 5–10 times; repeat with each fingertip in turn.

5. **Medial hand strengthener**. With your upper arm by your side, your elbow bent to a right angle and your palm facing upwards, grip a squash ball or similar soft object with your fourth and fifth fingers; squeeze gently, while keeping your thumb and other fingers relaxed. 5–10 times. *Variation: repeat with your elbow straight and your arm held at different angles from your body.*

6. **Grip strengthener**. Tense your hand round a soft ball, rolled towel or similar suitable object which fits into your hand; grip as hard as you can for a count of 5, then relax. 3–6 times. *Variations: a) use different types of grip exerciser; b) practise gripping with your elbow bent and your hand palm up, down and sideways; c) repeat with your elbow straight and your arm held at different angles from the shoulder.*

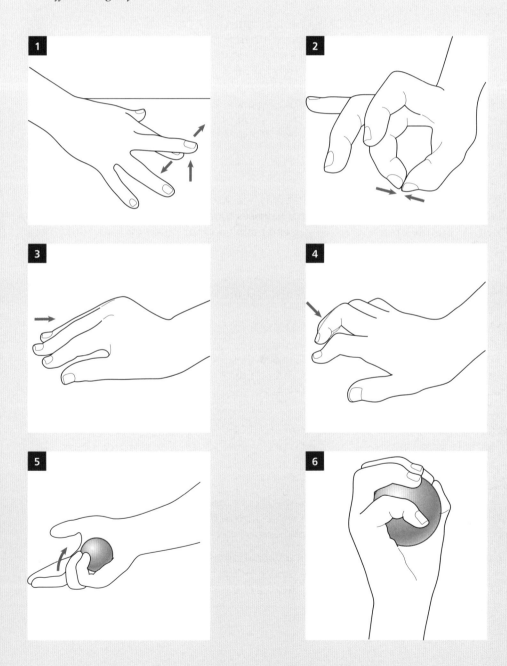

Wrist and hand stretching and mobilizing exercises

1. **Prayer stretch**. With your hands just in front of your chest, fingers straight and pointing upwards, press your palms together; keeping your palms in contact with each other, gently move your hands vertically downwards as far as you can; hold for a count of 6, then relax. 5–10 times.

2. **Wrist flexor stretch**. With your hands held forwards in front of your chest, fingers straight and pointing forwards, press your palms together; keeping your palms in contact with each other, draw your hands back towards your body and press your upper arms and elbows forwards slightly; hold for a count of 6, then relax. 5–10 times.

3. **Wrist extensor stretch**. With your arm forward so that your palm faces your body and your forearm is horizontal just in front of you, use your other hand to bend the fingers and wrist of your hand towards your forearm, stretching the back of the wrist and hand; hold for a count of 6, then relax. 5–10 times. *Variation: turn the hand downwards and repeat.*

4. **Wrist mobilizer**. With your arms by your sides, elbows bent to right angles and palms facing downwards, flick your hands up and down alternately at the wrists as fast as you can, keeping your arms still. 10–20 times.

5. **Finger stretches**. Put one hand palm down on a flat surface, and use the other hand to lift each finger in turn upwards and backwards as far as is comfortable, stretching the palm and flexor tendons; hold for a count of 6, then relax. 5–10 times.

6. **Thumb stretch inwards**. With your elbow bent to a right angle, hand and fingers forwards and straight, and your palm facing inwards so that your thumb is on top, use your other hand to bend your thumb and stretch it gently across your palm; hold for a count of 6, then relax. 5–10 times.

7. **Thumb stretch outwards**. Place your thumb and index finger on a flat surface, with your hand vertical, palm facing outwards; gently press downwards to separate your thumb from your fingers slightly; hold for a count of 6, then relax. 5–10 times.

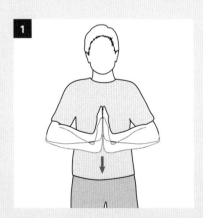
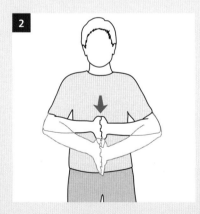

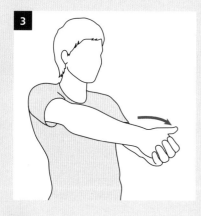

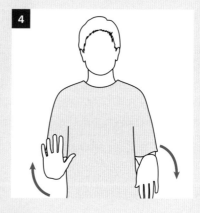

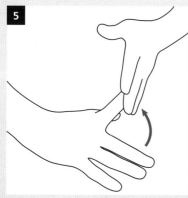

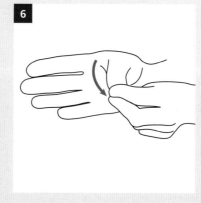

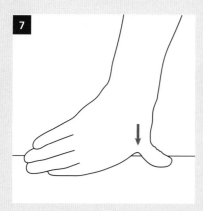

Advanced wrist and hand strengthening exercises

1. **Wrist and finger extension strengthener**. Sit, stand or kneel, resting your forearm on a support, with your elbow bent, hand free over the edge of the support, and palm down; with your fingers as straight as possible, lift your hand upwards from the wrist, keeping your forearm still; slowly reverse the movement. 5–10 times.

2. **Wrist extension strengthener**. Repeat exercise 1 gripping a light weight in your hand.

3. **Wrist and hand flexion strengthener**. Sit, stand or kneel, with your forearm resting on a support, elbow bent, hand free over the edge of the support and palm up; curl your fingers and bend your wrist to bring your hands upwards, keeping your forearm still; slowly reverse the movement. 5–10 times.

4. **Wrist flexion and grip strengthener**. Repeat exercise 3 gripping a light weight in your hand.

5. **Wrist abduction strengthener**. Sit, stand or kneel with the inner (medial) edge of your forearm resting on a support, hand slightly downwards over the edge of the support and your thumb uppermost; keeping the fingers straight and leading with the thumb, lift your hand vertically upwards into wrist abduction, keeping your forearm still; slowly reverse the movement. 5–10 times. Progress by holding a light weight, stick or racket in your hand.

6. **Wrist adduction strengthener**. Lying on your stomach on the edge of a bed, with your arm straight and wrist supported, place your hand slightly downwards over the side, fingers straight and little finger uppermost; leading with the little finger, raise the hand upwards (into wrist adduction), keeping the forearm still; slowly reverse the movement. 5–10 times. Progress by holding a light weight in your hand.

7. **Advanced grip strengthener**. Use a grip exerciser with increasing resistance.

8. **Hand dexterity**. Sitting with your elbow bent and your hand facing upwards, hold two golf balls or Chinese iron balls (make sure there is something soft for the balls to land on in case you drop them at first); rotate the balls around your hand, first anticlockwise then clockwise, using your fingers and thumbs to keep them apart. Do this little and often.

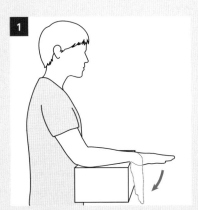

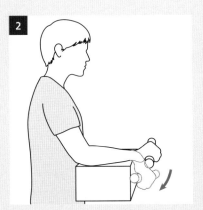

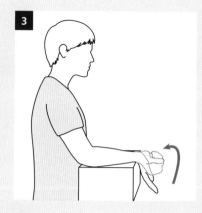

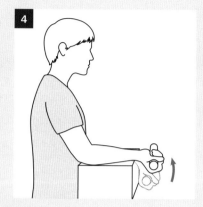

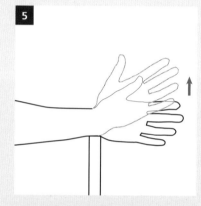

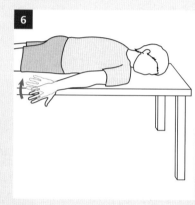

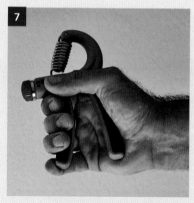

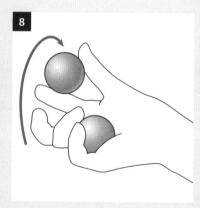

Final Recovery

Your injury has healed when you no longer have any pain. Your rehabilitation is complete when you have regained full strength and movement. The final stage of recovery includes dynamic exercises which can be incorporated into fitness training according to the needs of your sport, and a gradual return to your sport. You should keep doing daily protective rehabilitation exercises indefinitely, even after recovery.

Planning your fitness programme

It is best to work on your fitness with a coach or trainer. Your programme should be varied and progressive, and should allow days off for rest and recovery. You should avoid doing repetitive training such as running, cycling or skipping on consecutive days. A concentrated fitness block can be done once or twice a year and should cover a set period, which can be four to twelve weeks. If you are a competitor, your fitness training should be organized so that it does not interfere with your competition programme.

Body balance

Whatever your level, work on the whole body, not just the parts you need for your sport. Body balance is an important part of injury prevention. Always do more exercises, repetitions or sets for your weakest areas. Many sports develop parts of the body to the detriment of others. If you have strong legs from running or soccer, you should work especially on your trunk and arms. Shadow practice using the non-dominant side is a good way to counteract the one-sidedness of racket games or fencing.

The warm-up and cool-down

A warm-up prepares the body for activity by increasing your blood flow and improving mobility. It has never been shown to give particular protection against injury: most intrinsic injuries happen late on in a session or match, and are linked to fatigue or relative dehydration rather than cold muscles.

The warm-up can include stretching exercises, ballistic mobilizing exercises, some dynamic aerobic activities, some strengthening work, and some skill practices specific to your sport. In cold conditions you need to pay special attention to your hands and feet. When preparing for competition it can be helpful to include a short period of mental focussing on skills or tactics. I recommend gentle passive stretching first, followed by the other elements, and ending with more passive stretching when your body tissues are warm.

The cool-down, or warm-down, can help to prevent stiffness after strenuous exercise, and so might help prevent injuries. It is usually shorter than the warm-up, and consists primarily of stretching, together with some dynamic movements and gentle aerobic exercise.

Final-phase dynamic leg exercises

1. **Pelvic lift 'running'**. Lie on your back with your knees bent, hips off the floor; keeping your hips up, straighten each knee in turn as quickly as possible, kicking your foot upwards. 20–30 times.

2. **Cross-legged stand-ups**. Sit on a chair with knees parallel and one foot crossed over the other; without using your arms, stand up quickly straightening your knees fully, then sit down again with control. 5–10 times. Repeat reversing the crossed position of your feet.

3. **Alternate leg thrusts**. Crouch down to put your hands flat on the floor, with your fingers forwards; resting on your hands, kick one leg backwards, then forwards as you kick the other leg backwards. 10–20 times in quick succession.

4. **Squat thrusts**. Crouch down and balance your weight on your hands and toes, with your elbows and knees straight; resting on your hands, bring your knees up towards your chest in a horizontal jump, then quickly reverse the movement to kick your legs straight out behind you. 5–20 times without stopping.

5. **Calf and arm raises**. Standing with your feet slightly apart, with weights on your wrists or in your hands, go up on your toes and lift your arms sideways, keeping your knees and elbows straight; slowly reverse the movement. 5–20 times.

6. **Bench astride jumps**. Standing astride a bench 21–31 centimetres (8–12 inches) high, jump up to place both feet on the bench, then jump down to put your feet on the floor on either side of the bench. 5–20 times. Variation: jump up to touch your heels together above the bench, landing with your feet on either side of the bench.

7. **Squat jumps**. Stand with one foot slightly in front of the other; jump down to touch your hands to the floor, then spring up changing your foot position in the air, so that you land with the back foot in front. 5–20 times in quick succession.

8. **Burpees**. From standing, squat down quickly to put your hands flat on the floor; resting your weight on your hands, kick both legs backwards straightening your knees, bend your knees in a horizontal jump, then jump upwards straightening your knees in the air. 5–20 times in quick succession.

9. **Skip**. Use a skipping rope, first with both feet together, then alternate feet. 20–50 skips.

10. **Chest jumps**. From standing, jump upwards and bend your knees, bringing them as close to your chest as you can. 5–20 times without stopping.

11. **Shuttle runs**. Sprint to a set point, touch the ground, and sprint back to the start. 10–30 times. Variations: a) set the markers in different directions; b) number the markers and have an assistant call out which point you have to sprint to.

12. **Hop**. Hop forwards, sideways and backwards. 5–30 hops in each direction.

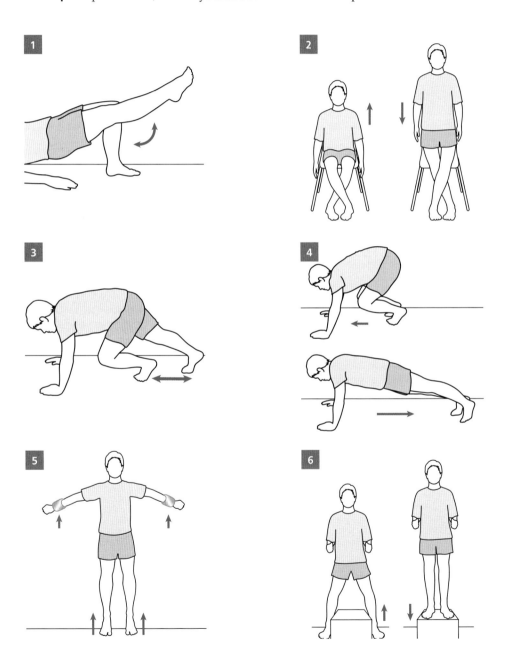

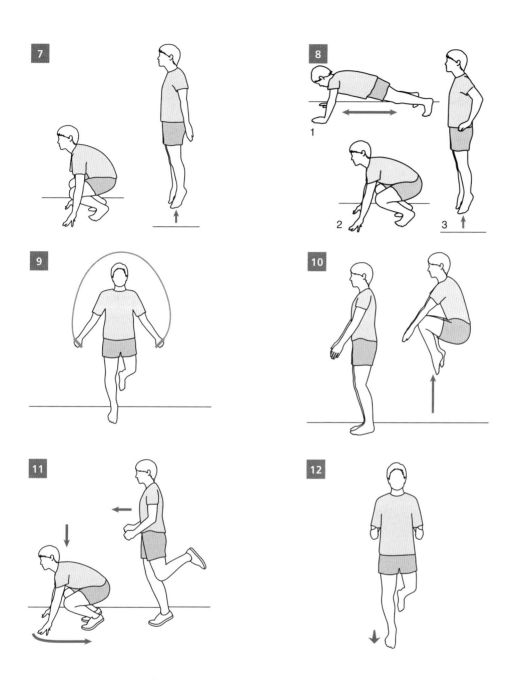

Final-phase dynamic arm exercises

1. **Lats pull-downs**. Use a lats machine to pull a weight downwards, keeping your back straight and head up. (If the machine uses a cord system, your hands should come down in front of you, not behind your neck.) 5–15 times.

2. **Press-ups**. Lie on your stomach with your hands level with your shoulders and palms down on the floor; push on your hands to straighten your elbows and lift your body up, so that you balance on your hands and feet; reverse the movement with control. 3–15 times.

3. **Chins**. Using a bar high enough for your body and legs to be off the ground, grip the bar and bend your elbows to lift your body up, keeping your hips extended; reverse the movement with control. 3–15 times. Variations: a) place your hands palms forwards facing away from your body, then backwards; b) place your arms at different angles so that your hands are further from each other or closer together.

4. **Sit-lifts**. Sit on a bench or wide chair, with your hands palms down on the bench just in front of your hips; lean forwards slightly and press down on your hands to lift your bottom off the support; reverse the movement with control. 3–15 times.

5. **Triceps dips**. Using a triceps dip machine, press down on your hands, straightening your elbows from the bent position. 3–15 times. Alternatively, use parallel bars off the ground: keeping your trunk vertical, grip the bars with your hands, bend your elbows with control to let your body glide downwards, then straighten your elbows quickly to raise yourself upwards. Variations: a) with hips and knees bent; b) with thighs vertical and knees bent.

6. **Backward press-ups**. Sit on the floor with your legs straight and your hands on the floor behind you, palms down; lift your pelvis up so that you rest on your hands and heels; bend your elbows with control to bring your body downwards, keeping your trunk in line; straighten your elbows quickly to lift your body up. 3–15 times.

7. **L-sits**. Sit on the floor with your legs straight in front of you and your hands palms down flat on the floor beside you, just in front of your hips; straighten your elbows, pressing down on your hands to lift your trunk and legs off the floor, keeping your legs straight and hips at right angles; slowly reverse the movement. 3–15 times.

8. **Side-raises, arm extended**. Lie on your side; keeping your arm straight place your hand on the floor under your shoulder, palm down, fingers pointing away from your body; lift your hips up to rest your weight on your hand and the side of your foot; reverse the movement with control. 3–15 times on each side.

9. **Inclined pulls to low bar**. Set the bar so that you can just reach it with your hands when you lie on the floor under it; keeping your trunk in line, grip the bar and bend your elbows so that you lift your body up and balance on your heels; reverse the movement with control. 5–15 times.

10. **Super side-raises**. Lie on your side, with your elbow bent so that your shoulder is off the floor; lift your hips upwards so that your weight is on your elbow, forearm and the side of your foot; move your upper arm and leg upwards and downwards 3–10 times; lower your hips and relax. 5–15 times on each side.

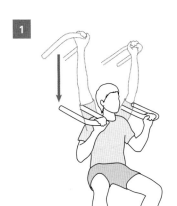

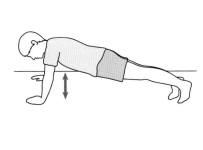

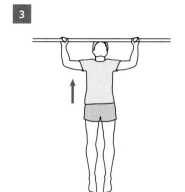

3

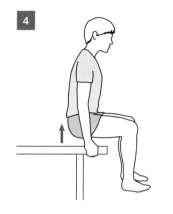

4

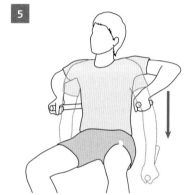

5

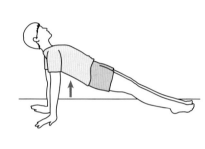

6

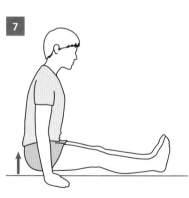

7

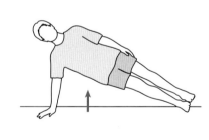

8

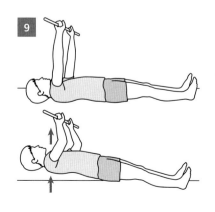

9

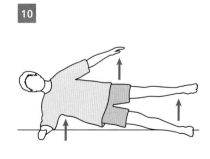

10

Return to sport

Your return to sport should be carefully graded. Scale down your practice if you have any recurrence of your injury symptoms.

Space out any kind of repetitive training or skills practice. This is especially important if you are recovering from an overuse injury such as a stress fracture. Whatever your sport, start with one session per week for the first three to four weeks, two sessions in the second month, three in the third, building up to four in the fourth. These sessions should be balanced by different types of training and exercise relating to your sport and for general fitness.

For one-sided sports like tennis, golf, fencing or throwing events, vary your sessions. If you are a runner, you can run on any surface when you restart, although a mixture is best. Try changing direction, doing short bursts sideways and backwards as well as forwards. Build up your distance in gradual stages.

Despite the commonly held view that you need to practise or train every day to be a top performer, it is better to allow days off each week, and regular periods off training and competing during the year. If you do that, you reduce the risks of staleness, overfatigue and injury, and the chances are your performance will be the better for it.

Index